The Deep Massage Book

How to Combine Structure and Energy in Bodywork

by

David Lauterstein

Illustrations by Christy Krames, M.A.

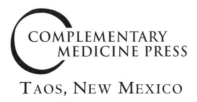
COMPLEMENTARY
MEDICINE PRESS

TAOS, NEW MEXICO

The Deep Massage Book

How to Combine Structure and Energy in Bodywork

David Lauterstein

© Complementary Medicine Press 2011

Library of Congress Cataloging-in-Publication Data

Lauterstein, David.
  The deep massage book : how to combine structure and energy in bodywork / David Lauterstein.
      p. ; cm.
  Includes bibliographical references and index.
  ISBN 978-0-9673034-8-2 (pbk. : alk. paper)
  I. Title.
  [DNLM: 1. Massage. 2. Musculoskeletal Manipulations--methods. WB 537]

615.8'22--dc23

2012000037

Published by
Complementary Medicine Press
Taos, New Mexico, USA
Distributed by Redwing Book Company
202 Bendix Drive, Taos NM 87571
www.redwingbooks.com

Library of Congress Number: 2012000037
International Standard Book Number (ISBN): ISBN 978-0-9673034-8-2

Printed in the United States of America   2 3 4 5 6 7 8 9

An absolute masterpiece! Written by a true master of this ancient craft; and a joy to read.

The great bodywork pioneer Ida P. Rolf described her work as "a series of principles that leaves behind it a trail of techniques." I cannot think of a better way to explain David Lauterstein's seamless way of presenting the principles of his Deep Massage method and the precise and innovative techniques that are organically birthed from them. Part poet, part philosopher of healing, and part master clinician, David—and his new text—comprise an invaluable resource to all sincere students of bodywork and manual therapy.

At the heart of this fine book is music. David Lauterstein—a voice of deep experience—sings the octave of the body's chakras to create a melody of deep-tissue protocols, bathed in the harmony of rich therapeutic contact, steadied by the bass tones of bodywork's place in our unfolding human story.

Finally, a book that explores the dimensions of touch through philosophy, psychology, structure, energy, and solid technique has been published! In *The Deep Massage Book*, David dares to use a holistic approach to define deep massage through logic, careful description, and the powerful link of touch to structure and energy. This book is a welcome addition to essential bodywork literature and is a must read for all students and practitioners. Well done, David!

David Lauterstein shares decades of dedication to the art and science of massage. The book is a reflection of the energy and structure of its subject. It is inviting; it communicates with clarity and assurance; it sings its wisdom from its roots. It extends the boundaries of our knowledge, enabling us to learn, with humanity, about our humanity. This is a very different kind of massage book—but then Deep Massage is a very different kind of massage.

Dedication

To my Mother and Father
> Thank you for inspiring me with art, science, and the hope for a better world.

To my Godmother, Millie Barry
> Thank you for your love, kindness, joy, and soul.

To Herbert Brun
> Thank you for your rigorous teaching of composition, both human and musical.

To my first massage teacher, Bob King
> Thank your for your mentoring, inspiration and lifelong friendship.

To Daniel Blake, the founder of Structural Bodywork
> Thank you for your teaching.

To Fritz Smith, M.D.
> Great teacher and friend, thank you for the gift of Zero Balancing.

To John Conway and the staff, faculty, and students of Lauterstein-Conway Massage School
> Thank you for twenty-five years of growth and learning.

To all my bodywork friends in England and the U.S. – Zanna Heighton, Pam Geggus, Clive Taylor, Jeff Lennard, Alan Hext, Nancy Dail, and others
> Thank you for your many years of support and friendship.

To Paul Brown
> Thank you for being my consiglière and friend all these years.

To my daughter, Katja
> Thank you for your vision and for being who you are.

To my son, Jake
> Thanks for helping during a critical time with the book, and for your enthusiastic dedication to your path.

To Julie Lauterstein
> Love of my life, thank you for being who you are and doing what you do to make every day a blessing.

Preface

The practice of "Deep Massage," like all approaches, is fed by many rivers of influence. To give credit to and to fully acknowledge each of these would entail a book unto itself. What follows is the essential background.

The first thirty years of my life were spent mostly playing guitar and studying philosophy and art, particularly music. I studied aesthetics, folk music, rock and roll, Indian music, and classical Western composition (BA, U of Illinois, 1972.) Thus, some of the earliest ideas that found a home in Deep Massage flowed from my thoughts and experiences of how it is that art has the power to move people deeply.

I began to transition to bodywork in the early '70s, first from personal interest and by 1977 as a profession. I was fascinated by the mind-body connection and saw it as a route—more direct than music—for people to attain higher levels of health, happiness, and inspiration in their lives.

My first bodywork mentor, Bob King, founder of the Chicago School of Massage Therapy, showed me, among many other things, that whatever tension I maintained in my own bodymind would be felt by clients. So he quickly helped me see that the route for the client's healing also held true for the therapist.

In 1982-83, I studied with Rolfer Daniel Blake, who had a developed his own outgrowth of Rolfing called "Structural Bodywork," in which I became certified. Daniel was a brilliant anatomy and bodywork instructor who had developed a remarkable system for analyzing muscular tension patterns involved in structural misalignments—postural kinesiology.

Thereafter I began teaching anatomy and deep tissue massage at the Chicago School of Massage Therapy. Through interaction with these first students, I was naturally inspired to develop a method for conveying the art as well as the science of bodywork.

In 1982-83, I also studied Craniosacral Therapy, with early students of Dr. John Upledger. Cranial work clearly showed that less is more—sometimes no pressure at all can have a deeper effect than the considerable pressure I had been using in structural bodywork.

It was at that point that I changed the name of my therapeutic approach from "Deep Tissue" to "Deep Massage." I had come to realize that we weren't working simply on tissues. We weren't simply effecting the release of the muscles and fascia. We were working with the whole person with the aim of affecting him or her in a deeply positive way.

In 1986, I began studying with Dr. Fritz Smith, MD, the founder of Zero Balancing. Through practicing and teaching Zero Balancing, I received a language and heightened awareness of how to convey, in my practice and teaching, the precise way to connect with structure and energy simultaneously. I was certified as a practitioner in 1993 and as a teacher of Zero Balancing in 1996.

I have taught the Lauterstein Method of Deep Massage since 1982 throughout the U.S. and in England. In 1989, I launched a massage and bodywork school in Austin, Texas with my business partner and co-instructor, John Conway. It is here, at the Lauterstein-Conway Massage School, where we have further developed this work and trained over 2,000 therapists.

It is remarkable that one can describe so many years of learning and growth in just a few paragraphs! Similarly, the contributions of teachers and friends can be put in a few words even though they resonate through one's entire life—just as the right, simple touch at the perfect moment can change everything.

A Note on the Structure of this Book

The Deep Massage Book has essentially three parts.

Part One, which comprises the first four chapters, presents the essential science and theory of Deep Massage.

Part Two alternates inspiring philosophical chapters with chapters on imaginative anatomy and techniques. The philosophical chapters each explore one of seven distinct dimensions of touch. They fully elaborate the basic theories of Deep Massage into a philosophy of touch.

The technical chapters have exacting descriptions and beautiful illustrations to help you learn very clear "fulcrums" for working with body structure and energy. For the artwork, special thanks are due my collaborator, Christy Krames, a master of medical illustration, whom I was fortunate enough to discover here in my hometown of Austin, Texas.

Part Three looks at how to combine these theories and techniques in individualized session design. It further explores how the renaissance of touch we are experiencing can contribute to changes desperately needed in our world today.

Amongst the clear theory, the precise techniques, and the inspiration of the philosophy presented herein, my hope is that readers, therapists, and everyone they touch will have their work and life greatly enhanced through the unique principles and practice of Deep Massage.

Acknowledgements

Special thanks to Naomi Shihab Nye for permission to reprint an excerpt from her poem, *Two Countries* (p. 149); to Richard Tillinghast for permission to reprint *If You Love the Body* (p. 157); and to Elliot Greene for permission to reprint his haiku (p. 29).

Table of Contents

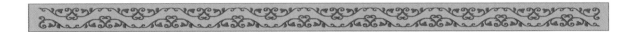

Part One

Hands make the world each day.

— Pablo Neruda

Deep Massage
and the Renaissance of Touch

A Renaissance took place in Europe in the 15th and 16th centuries. We have all studied it, and thousands of books are devoted to the subject. Today, we find ourselves in the midst of another renaissance, one predicted by the futurist John Naisbitt in his book, *Megatrends.* He spoke of the coming world as one of "High Tech, High Touch."

The rise of High Tech and its spellbinding world of virtual reality has become a pervasive aspect of contemporary society. At the same time, this renaissance of connecting with sight and sound has been accompanied by a renaissance of touch. Thus the rise of "High Touch" and its corresponding commitment to the heightened experience of *actual* reality is a renaissance that is equally newsworthy and of potentially greater significance.

The most profound of our senses and the earliest to develop, touch is at the forefront of one of the truly remarkable developments of our age. The discovery hovering in the margins of mainstream awareness is that touch is quite possibly the leading edge for the next step in our cultural evolution.

It is no accident that there has been far more proliferation of touch therapies in the last twenty years than at any other time in world history. Nor is it any particular methodology of touch that is singularly powerful — be it Swedish massage, Zero Balancing, Reiki, Craniosacral Therapy, or Rolfing. These all are modalities pointing us back to the source of our power — *our selves* and the life force we embody.

Setting aside the claims of the various therapeutic modalities, what is most powerful is the transformative power of touch, allowing us to fully encounter the truth of our aliveness, to restore our sense of deep joy, to awaken to and exult with tender touch in the beauty of being human. Touch connects us at many levels. Touch wakens us from the illusory world of happiness marketed to us through virtual reality and the accumulation of material goods, the kind of happiness that takes no inner work. *Touch entails the medium of actual reality.*

The hunger for what is real in a culture of alienation is the greatest hunger of all. Touch is a fundamental way to satisfy this hunger for the real. How can we optimize this power? How can we best use it to help in actualizing our vision of a world that values and cultivates real life? How can we ensure the expanded growth and cultural influence of the high art and science of touch?

Deep Massage is a way to understand and cultivate this quality of touch. At the same time, Deep Massage is clinically effective and uniquely revitalizing. It has met with success because humankind is badly in need of solutions to stress-related disease and to the deep sense of disconnectedness that is a byproduct of modern culture. Deep Massage is a natural outgrowth of the many innovations in body and mind therapies occurring today, arising from a new understanding of human structure and energy.

Until this past century our understanding of anatomical structure was based on a compression model. It was thought that the body was supported by the bones resting on top of one another, just as columns support one another in a building. The muscles were viewed strictly as elements of movement.

The foundations of modern structural bodywork and Deep Massage formed with the realization that the bones themselves are held in position largely by the muscles and their associated connective tissues, called "fasciae." As early as the 19th century, Andrew Taylor Still, the founder of osteopathy, recognized fascia's role in health. A century later Ida Rolf, the founder of Rolfing ("Structural Integration"), articulated both a theory and practice based solidly on this model.

Similarly, and in the same era of time and culture, Buckminster Fuller, a visionary architect, writer, and thinker of the mid-20th century, studied the interrelationship of form and function and coined the term "tensegrity" to describe their interplay in architecture as well as throughout nature. He observed that the hard members in a structural system are supported and positioned by the soft members. Think of how tent poles are actually held in place by the tensions in the canvas and guy wires. Thus, just as the soft members of the tent position the tent poles, the positioning of bones, and thus our overall alignment, is largely determined by the tensing and lengthening of our muscles and their fascia.

Consequently, these powerful conceptual breakthroughs opened up a whole new role for bodywork. If muscles and their associated connective tissues were understood as the primary element in determining the body's alignment and movement, then massage therapy would hold a central position with regard to the health of the human structure—perhaps even a central position with regard to human culture. Ida Rolf deeply valued this aspect of bodywork, considering it critical to the furtherance of human evolution.

We have evolved from forward-leaning apes toward erectness and the promise of deep balance potential within the human form. In this sense the attainment of our vertical destiny appears to be a prerequisite to physical health as well as perhaps a foundation for the emotional, spiritual, and mental health of the fully embodied human.

The Muscular and Fascial Basis for Change

The basis for muscular change lies partly within the fasciae, the living connective tissues that help determine the muscles' form. Fascia is found everywhere in the body. It covers each bone, where it is called periosteum. It covers and invests the entire peripheral nervous system, surrounding the whole nerve as the epineurium, each bundle of neurons as the perineurium, and each individual neuron as the endoneurium.

The outermost layers of the arteries, lymphatic vessels, and digestive tubes are made of fasciae. Where it surrounds the brain and spinal cord it is known as the meninges. Where it connects the bones it is called ligament. And, of course, remarkably similar to the neural structure, fascia covers and invests the muscles, surrounding the whole muscle as epimysium, muscle bundles as perimysium, and individual muscle cells as the endomysium. At either end of the muscle these connective tissue layers continue beyond the muscle fibers and are then named tendons. Fascia is an extremely complex, three-dimensional spider-webbing that gives the whole and each part of the body its shape and its relationship in space to every other part.

Fascia has other functions as well. It acts protectively, like a second skin. It has immune and regenerative functions in case of disease and injury. It is also a conductor of piezo-electric current. Some texts refer to fascia chemically as liquid crystal!

Thus we can begin to understand the excitement and profundity of Ida Rolf's answer to a reporter's question of why she worked with fascia: "Because that's what I can get my hands on!" As we see now, fascia is, along with water itself, a substance through which it is possible to address the entire human being. Touch, combined with deep knowledge of the form and function of fascia, has the potential to transform the whole person.

Fascia has one more remarkable property that makes hands-on therapies especially powerful. The word for this quality is "thixotrophic." The chemical nature of a thixotrophic substance is such that any increase in its activity results in it becoming more fluid. Other thixotrophic substances include some clays in the earth, synovial fluid in the joints, and even cornstarch and toothpaste. When these are stirred, shaken, squeezed, or moved in any way, they become more fluid.

Fascia is composed largely of a ground substance, called hyaluronic acid, housing occasional protein fibers, most often collagen. It is the hyaluronic acid that is thixotrophic, such that the moment we press into the body it immediately starts becoming more fluid. The heat of the therapist's hands also increases this activity and thus the fluidity within the tissue, especially in more congested areas where circulation is impeded. The energy of the therapist's touch, whether we define it electrochemically or psychologically, also plays a role in increasing fluidity.

The human hand, acting in concert with the heart, mind, and spirit, is arguably the most sophisticated tool in the known physical universe. With its pressure and warmth, guided by intelligence, care, and inspiration, we can work with muscles and fascia, literally remodeling the human form and dramatically altering each and every human function.

The Role of the Nervous System

Connected to the fasciae and muscles is one more element that further speaks to the power of bodywork. Embedded within the muscle and fasciae are nerves referred to as proprioceptors. These nerves are designed to monitor, in concert with the brain, our every movement and interaction with the environment. Asleep and awake, they register the amount of pressure of the things that contact us.

Proprioceptors also track the length or tension in each muscle. Using this information, the brain creates its perception of the body—its shape, movement, and posture.

The brain constructs the experience of the body, the relative size and position of body parts, and their relationship with respect to one another in space.

Notice how peculiar it feels when your foot "goes to sleep." Your balance is completed affected. The proprioceptors, temporarily deprived of oxygen, are not getting their messages to your brain, so you effectively lose the clear experience of having a foot! Accordingly, muscles may be even more important as sensing organs than as organs of movement. Without their neural role, we cannot experience where a body part is or how it is shaped. And without the experienced information of how we are structured, we cannot coherently move.

Of course, balancing the muscles' sensory role is their motor role, and here as well the nervous system is intimately interwoven with the muscles. Nerves run to each group of muscle fibers. Muscles contract or relax only in response to messages from the nervous system. The musculofascial guywires and fabrics within our tensegrity system do not have set lengths, but at any moment, they can alter their lengths in response to the varying flow of neural input.

Chronically tense muscles are only so in response to neural stimulation. Relaxation, therefore, is not initiated by the muscles themselves, but is effected in the muscle when the nervous input ceases. Contrary to the usual notion of relaxation being elicited mechanically by massage through rubbing the muscles, muscular relaxation is actually caused by the therapist's touch changing the nervous system!

How can we do this? Massage the nervous system? In some respect this is the question addressed by this book—because when we know how to contact and change the nervous system, we have our hands on proprioception, and through it, the whole world of body image and touch associations.

Consider that touch, being the earliest sense to develop in the embryo, influences our fundamental assumptions about the world and our place in it. When we focus our touch on the muscles and connective tissues, we have maximum leverage with respect to these formative assumptions. In a completely literal sense, we have in our hands the very basis for human evolution. Yes, we get our hands on fascia. Yet suddenly, through the nervous system, the existential arena in which massage operates becomes not merely physical structure, but the whole texture of consciousness, emotions, memories, and dreams.

With the same skill and inspiration as any great artist, we use our knowledge and our hands as the tools to help align and revitalize human beings. Our medium is not paint or musical tones. It is the structure and energy of the human being!

The Miracle of Human Structure and Energy

Modern medicine has primarily involved the study and practice of attending to the physical aspect of the person. Anatomists have looked at the biological things, named them, and identified their locations. Medicine has focused on diseases or injuries, diagnosis, and treatment. Such careful attention has yielded vast rewards: we have effective cures for many diseases that once were lethal; we have witnessed the virtual elimination of smallpox, measles, polio; we benefit from incredible advances in surgeries of all kinds, including arthroscopic breakthroughs.

Daily, these advances contribute to millions of lives being healthier and to increased longevity. Many of us are alive today as a result of modern medicine. All homage paid to its life-sustaining power!

At the same time that Western medicine has successfully treated the physical body, it has not been particularly innovative with regard to the treatment of the individual. I recall, for example, a physical therapist telling me, "I'm seeing four knees this morning." Western medicine does not essentially take into account the feelings, thoughts, spirit, or soul of the patient. It pays attention to structure primarily, with little attention paid to energy.

"Energy," for our purposes, refers to anything not strictly physical. Whereas structure relates to matter and particles, and is solid, visible, and tangible, energy relates to waves, vibrations, movement, and, in humans, the epiphenomena of sensation, awareness, self-consciousness, beliefs, emotions, and spirit.

What remains problematic is two-fold. First, a medicine that ignores the person will tend to fail at treating chronic problems because these often have to do with people's behavior rather than an identifiable pathogen. Second, a medicine that ignores the personhood of the patient will not promote therapeutic trust. Patients whose emotional state is ignored become resentful, even though the disease treatment may go well!

This undoubtedly contributes to why medical malpractice suits are common. If a medicine does not relate to the feeling, thinking, and spiritual side of the person, it can seriously compromise the healthy relationship between doctor and patient. Leaving energy out of the equation is itself a cause of "dis"-ease, in the sense that relationships where trust does not fully exist lack "ease." This, in turn, ultimately has physiological and social consequences.

We may indeed consider the separation of structure from energy as a cultural wound or epidemic. A medicine or a society that regards people as objects is one that leaves the worlds of feeling, thought, and spirit to the vicissitudes of chance. This describes, certainly in some respects, the world we find ourselves in today. Education teaches children how to manipulate symbols and facts, but continues to avoid issues pertaining to the energetic world—

beliefs, emotions, ethics, spirit. Religion, wielding diminished authority for many, no longer takes up the slack.

Western science bases itself on empiricism—it looks closely at what is observable and draws scientific conclusions from it. But in humans, emotion is an important part of what _is_! It follows that any science that ignores emotions is simply sloppy science. In people there is matter and there is also energy. To speak of life without either is senseless. Leaving discussions of energy out of our examination of structure is like leaving meaning out of a discussion of language.

That scientists have separated structure from energy and paid the physical aspect undue attention is not their fault. It is the vestige of a pervasive cultural phenomenon traceable to the philosophical problem called "mind-body dualism" that has haunted Western thought throughout its history. We have developed a primarily materialistic culture. In a materialistic world the ability to possess things is often associated, however naively, with happiness. Indeed, the worship of objects, from the golden calf of the Bible to the idolatry of the computer, forms an important strand in our history. As with most either-or conundrums, however, the obvious solution is "both-and."

The Evolution of Structure

Structure is miraculous. How remarkable that all the myriad forms of matter exist — beginning with the complex structure of the atom, then moving on to the countless combinations of molecules, the living cell, and multi-cellular organisms in the full ecstatic variety of plant and animal forms, all the way to the unimaginable vastness of the planets and stars.

The evolution of structure is a thrilling tale written in the very matter of life. We are, in every cell, tissue, and organ, the result of the trials, errors, and successes of trillions of creatures! We are the result of struggles so many and ceaseless that it seems awe is the only appropriate response to the evolved form we have taken. Each living thing embodies uniquely the structural solutions of countless other living and non-living objects that have preceded us. In our structure — as in our energy — we are the inheritors of the miracle of evolutionary learning.

This would be enough! Yet with a change of focus we see the spark that quickens matter to movement. From a simple vibration, to electricity, to a waveform, to the energy we call life, to sensation, willed movement, emotion, consciousness, and, uniquely in humans, to the ability to reflect on all this, nature becomes conscious of itself! All these again are energetic properties since they are not physical. They may presuppose having a brain and a particular biochemistry, but as phenomena they are clearly not structures. Although love will never be found under a microscope, perhaps nothing gives life more meaning.

Building from these energetic foundations, humans have further developed vast stores of belief and learning. Languages, music, scientific knowledge itself, philosophy, the entire realm of values, ethics, and spirit — these live as well under the aegis of energy.

It as if we were just now waking from a dream, one dating back to the prehistory of real healthcare. A medicine and culture that does not take feelings, ideas, spirit — the whole realm of energy — into account is still in the dark ages. In spite of all our material and technological progress, we are just commencing our commitment to work fully with the whole of what constitutes the human being. The renaissance stirs.

The Evolutionary Role of Touch

Energy is eternal delight.

—William Blake

Thus we move beyond the either-or of structure-energy dualism and begin our exploration of the vastly more real world of "both-and." Obviously, in the world of our experience, energy and structure are one. We do not have our body over here and our feelings in some other location. Like the vibrating air column within the structure of a flute, the music of life is essentially this interaction of structure and energy.

How can we amplify this into a living experience and not just a useful insight? Here touch reveals an even more emphatic reason for its pivotal role in our modern culture.

Touch bears a precious evolutionary secret with regard to structure and energy. Touch involves the contact of one physical structure with another. However—and this is vitally important—touch also involves the contact of one energy with another. Would you say you are being touched by the chair you sit on or by the floor as you walk? No. Touch requires energetic as well as structural contact. For it to be touch it must involve intentionality, that is, energy.

Herein lies an enormous secret.

Touch is the only medium in the known universe that simultaneously and consciously contacts both structure and energy. We can think, look, and hear. But these do not require direct physical contact with the object of our perception.

Touch, and touch alone, necessarily and simultaneously contacts energy as well as structure. People in our world suffer from the dominance of structural models and the disregard of energy—the body of the individual and the body politic is treated while the person and deeper human needs are often ignored.

It bears repeating: *touch, and touch alone, necessarily and simultaneously contacts energy as well as structure.* It is therefore the primary medium for healing this tragic cultural wound between energy and structure. When we are deeply touched, we experience the re-union of the self; we experience being wholly and simultaneously connected in body, mind, and spirit.

Now we begin to see in its full majesty the profound power supporting the current phenomenal growth of massage therapy and other bodywork forms! If touch is indeed the only medium that can consciously contact both energy and structure, then it offers a solution to what may be the most critical problem facing human civilization. The estrangement of energy and structure is resolved through the entwinement of structure and energy in touch.

Interface

All real living is meeting.

—Martin Buber

Looking more closely at touch, we notice it is not just random touch that heals. It is touch with a certain energetic and structural quality. Since it plays a pivotal role in our culture and in any enlightened approach to healthcare, it is important to look closely at how we can cultivate the structural and energetic integrity of our touch.

Massage therapists and other hands-on health professionals may spend hundreds of hours mastering various strokes and the choreography of hand and body positions necessary to perform them, yet relatively little time to developing the energetic aspects of touch. Optimally, we might just as rigorously cultivate the knowledge and practice of how to refine the energetics of touch. We can then develop and potentially master the fascinating practice of "psycho-mechanics" to the same level of competence as our mastery of body mechanics.

Taken together, psycho-mechanics and body mechanics help us answer how one person's energy and structure can most appropriately meet the energy and structure of another. Boundaries, both structural and energetic, have been usefully emphasized the last several years in bodywork and psychotherapy. Each living being has physical as well as energetic boundaries that need to be respected.

This means each touch, in addition to a certain quantifiable pressure, will have a distinctively sensed quality: nurturing, annoying, invasive, consoling, invigorating, creepy, unclear, soothing—there are literally infinite associations, miraculously evolved within our nervous systems, such that each touch evokes a unique sensory experience. Through our sensations each touch affects the whole world of associations and memories housed in key neural structures in the brain. From these places, the effects of the touch radiate out through every aspect of the person. A local touch has a global effect.

A touch that is just right is one that evokes the most positive psychological association and positive biological consequence. One assumption of Deep Massage is that touching which consciously respects structural and energetic boundaries will result in the most consistently clear, positive, and health-giving impact. The key to achieving this touch quality is "interface" or "working at interface."

To work at interface, you first learn to center yourself and pay conscious attention to what you doing so that you are consciously sensing as well as moving with your hands. Your energy as well as your physical structure is present in the contacting surface. Then, with your beginning touch, you mindfully add just enough force to sense your structure and energy meeting that of your client.

Structurally, this means applying pressure until you feel the beginning of resistance or tension within the body. Energetically, this means bringing your awareness to just this place where you meet. This is similar to meditation, in which one commonly brings awareness to a home base—a mantra, a place in the body, breathing. When working at interface, we bring this awareness precisely to where we meet.

Consciously feel the clarity of this meeting point. Do not imagine that your energies are blending, becoming one. Do not imagine that the client's energy is streaming into you or yours into them. Just make a clear interface with structure and energy, at the physical and sensory boundary—only then can two conscious beings experience a safe and clear and satisfying sense of being in touch.

Working at interface is a revelation in body therapies because it establishes a clear guideline for the choreography not just of the body, but of the mind-heart-spirit.

There is no greater miracle in the history of creation than the conscious meeting of one embodied soul with another.

Creating a Fulcrum

The primary operational tool in Deep Massage is the fulcrum. According to the *American Heritage Dictionary*, a fulcrum is "an agent, around, through, or by means of which vital powers are exercised." In the context of Deep Massage, a fulcrum is a touch experience through which the client mobilizes his or her own vital powers to amplify health. Any touch that consciously contacts both structure and energy with attention, care, and skill can become a fulcrum, facilitating healing for the client's structure and energy.

The language of touch is composed of significant movements of mind and matter. The concept of the fulcrum has contributed an initial grammar for healing touch. For a sentence to make sense it has to have at least a noun and verb, with other optional parts of speech, in a particular order. For touch to have significance and power we must make specific ordered movements with our physical structure and our energy. Just as a sentence uses parts of speech particularly arranged to make sense, the fulcrum uses "parts of touch" particularly arranged to facilitate bodymind change.

Deep Massage is about creating relationships, beginning with a healthier relationship to one's own body, mind, and spirit. It is equally about creating healthier relationships to other people and the world around us. Each relationship is an engagement. The steps of the fulcrum can be seen not only as "parts of touch" but also as the archetypal steps of engagement.

Consider, for example, how we make an acquaintance. First we see the person. Then, if we choose, we greet them. Then we converse and get to know them. As we talk we determine possible future directions. We need to spend a certain amount of time in conversation sensing if these directions are or could be fruitful. As we are talking we monitor for when it may be time to disengage. Finally we say goodbye, perhaps to meet again.

These same archetypal steps can be looked at using any relationship metaphor—visiting a house, driving a car, getting to know a new city, reading a book. We determine our focus; we approach it, get to know it, take action with respect to it, know when we are done and then move on. These steps—the articulate arrangements of the parts of touch in a fulcrum—are:

1) Centering
2) Taking out the looseness
3) Taking up the slack
4) Moving in a curve
5) Holding and Balancing—Sustaining the Gesture
6) Monitoring for change
7) Clearly disengaging

PRACTICAL EXPERIMENT — A HANDSHAKE

With a partner, exchange handshakes with and without structural and energetic clarity. Decide first who will be the giver and who the receiver.

Giver: Let your attention be elsewhere – for instance on what you ate for dinner last night. Thus distracted, grasp the receiver's hand as if you were about to shake it. Hold in this manner, with your attention elsewhere, for 3-5 seconds.

Receiver: Notice how this feels. Then, again with distraction, take the handshake up and down. Then clearly disengage.

Now have the same giver imagine that he is truly interested in meeting and getting to know the receiver. Then grasp the receiver's hand in this non-distracted manner in which you make contact with both your energy and your structure. Hold for 3-5 seconds. Take the handshake up and down. Clearly disengage.

Together discuss your experiences, as giver and as receiver. Then switch roles and repeat the exercise, and again discuss your experiences. Did you notice different emotions and bodily sensations with the different ways of touching? Did you notice your thinking or your spirit change?

Note the sensations experienced from the receiver's standpoint, being related to in these different ways. Note also the differences from the giver's standpoint of not energetically meeting the person vs. both structural and energetic engagement.

Centering

Centering — we attend to our body, mind, spirit, and heart so that our structure and energy are, as much as possible, present and balanced in our touch.

An ancient Chinese philosopher is credited with the famous saying that each journey, however long, begins with a single step. For massage therapists, this step is centering. Centering is the act of balancing in the body, mind, heart, and spirit. Physically it is generally a matter of not leaning too far forward, backward, or to either side. In this manner we work most gracefully, using gravity mostly for pressure, not effort. If we are grounded and buoyant, we feel good and balanced in our bodies as we work.

Mentally, centering involves a letting go of pre-inclinations, of pre-judgments, so that we approach the client with an open mind. In this way we prepare to truly receive the other person. We initiate the mysterious process of really endeavoring to understand someone else. Their representation in us cannot develop unless we approach them with openness. Think of it as a sort of open field in our mind in which our understanding of them can take root and grow.

Spiritually, centering involves having a sense of one's place in the universe. We cultivate humility. We are in no way better than the client, we simply embody some useful knowledge. We are not superior healing beings, we are an integral part of this amazing world, known and unknown. Spiritual centering involves clear self-awareness, free from making ourselves smaller or larger than we really are.

Neither do we diminish nor do we elevate the client: fully centered, we approach the person with respect and with sincere personal regard.

Centering ourselves in terms of the heart involves being aware of what we feel without judgment, comparisons, or the need to discharge the feeling. For instance, if I feel frustrated during a session, it is important to acknowledge it but not to judge myself or express it in my touch. Frustration may even be the source of some important information—it wouldn't exist if there weren't a reason for it.

Breathing is usually the best and simplest tool to simultaneously center oneself in all these realms. Breathing relaxes the body and the mind, soothes the emotions, and inspires us. It is said that breath is the bridge between matter and spirit.

Centering is a continual, life-long commitment. When I'm not centered, my energy and structure are out of sync. Therefore, for structurally and energetically integrative work, centering is the single most important activity. We center ourselves not just at the beginning of the session—for in the first step is embodied the entire journey. Centering continues throughout the session, and ideally throughout the course of our entire life. It sets the stage for everything else. Our whole life begins with our first breath, and each successive breath keeps the play alive. Centering is the foundation for all work that aims to balance structure and energy.

A self-secret of Deep Massage is this: in its practice, the therapist experiences centering increasingly more often. We get better at it as a mindbody skill. In this fashion, centering becomes more and more an integral part of our lives. This in turn contributes to a healthier, saner life and to lifelong learning. Deep Massage is a path for mindbody growth for the therapist as well as the client.

Taking out the Looseness

Taking out the looseness – we move into the physical body until we begin to touch the person and not just his or her body.

Returning to the handshake exercise, notice how it feels when you shake someone's hand and they respond with little pressure. We say it feels like a "dead fish." By this we express that touch does not feel fully alive or even human, until our touch is actively met. Conversely, when we feel someone pressing actively back and feel well met, we immediately begin to come to interface. Remember, interface is clearly contacting with structure and energy.

Structure, by definition, has a boundary. Taking out the looseness means to be contacted at the boundary. In bodywork we come across the precise boundaries of a person when we press in deeply enough to feel the shape of what's under the surface. We may for instance feel, without too much pressure, tension within soft tissue, like the feeling of stepping into a pool of water, reaching down with our feet to touch the bottom.

Energetically, when we touch and remain centered, the person senses our attention right where the touch is taking place. In this manner two awarenesses come into contact.

This is an evolutionary privilege we have—to be self-aware, to have sensations, to be capable of movement, and to be capable of consciously touching another being.

All these wonders are embodied in taking out the looseness.

Taking up the Slack

Taking up the slack – now each movement we make is clearly and strongly felt by the client.

Centering brings the therapist in touch with his or her own structure and energy. Taking out the looseness involves an introduction to the client's energy and structure. Taking up the slack entails full engagement.

In a handshake, notice how looseness is taken out in order to have any sense of contact. Pressing even more deeply, the slack is completely taken up when you feel clearly the outlines of the bones underlying the soft tissue. For example, when we press just deeply enough into someone's shoulder tension, they may say, "That's it! You've got it!" At that moment we have taken up the slack.

Specifically then:

1) We center our energy.

2) We take out the looseness by pressing just enough so that the client begins to feel engaged.

3) Taking up the slack, we press in further until the client feels fully and completely engaged.

In our society, hellos and goodbyes are often rushed. Yet the actions they accompany—coming together and separating—are two of the most powerful experiences in life. Taking up the slack is a step that reminds us to honor the process of actively entering the client's world of structure and energy. It recognizes the boundaries and steps of a healthy relationship, as in entering someone's home respectfully—we don't just walk in and go for the refrigerator! We center ourselves at the doorway, enter through the door (taking out the looseness), introduce ourselves, and are welcomed to enter and visit. Taking up the slack is having the courage and courtesy (note they both come from the root word for "heart") to respect the boundaries of the other person's world of structure and energy.

Buddhist teacher Thich Nhat Hanh has said, "The body is not only the temple, it is also the sage." By taking up the slack consciously and caringly, we explicitly recognize the sacredness of the bodily home, this temple, this sage.

Moving in a Curve

Moving in a curve – we follow the natural forms and energetic pathways of the body. Rather than being straight, the pathways of body and mind are curving, living pathways to be traveled with mindful curiosity and respect.

After the slack has been taken up, even our slightest movement is clearly felt by the client. Therefore, how we move is of vast importance. If the client senses a kind of automatic movement with no curiosity, we will jeopardize the energetic interface.

If we press too hard or back off and re-introduce too much looseness, we run a similar risk of losing our clear engagement. Of course, if we do not know our anatomy and move in directions irrelevant to the particular myofascial structures with which we are working, we can lose the structural aspect of the interface.

In nature, the shapes and lines of things are all more or less curved and irregular. Straight lines, on the other hand, are man-made abstractions, an insinuation of geometry. When we follow any structure in the body, it is important to be conscious of the unique curve we naturally follow. In this way, the client feels his or her nature is recognized and honored.

When we move in a curve, the client senses we are not moving mechanically. When we introduce a curve to our movements, however slight, the client will sense that we are proceeding with curiosity. Linearity, by contrast, communicates nonverbally that the therapist is on autopilot, performing the stroke with no attention given to the particularity of the person's form and energy.

Even physics says that the shortest distance between two points is a curve (since space itself is curved). In the curve lies a secret that helps us cure the client and keep ourselves free from the narrow, fictional world of linearity that our mental habits sometimes incline us toward.

In the movement, in the grammar of the fulcrum, non-linearity is necessary to create inquiring and meaningful touch.

Hold and Balance—Sustaining the Gesture

Holding the contact or sustaining the gesture— now that the fulcrum is "built," we allow the client open time to deeply experience it.

Meaning and healing require sustained relationship. For touch to have power it must be sustained, much as a handshake needs a satisfying structural and energetic duration. Once we begin moving in a curve—whether it be our curved fingers pressing into a tense place, or our loose fists beginning to follow the gently curving path of a long tendon—and continue to hold, we facilitate the experience of a single, sustained, and positive mindbody event.

The nature of a fulcrum is to provide a heightened experience of time and space within, around, and by means of which we balance. The step of holding/sustaining the gesture involves a kind of not-doing. We remain centered, having taken out the looseness in the body; the slack is taken up, and the movement begun. We add nothing—we just hold the point or sustain the gesture. During this time, as the therapist actively rests, the next step is naturally taken by the client.

As the therapist holds a point or sustains the gesture, he or she (and often the client as well) goes into a witness state or what the psychologist Thomas Gordon described as "active listening," in this case an active listening to the bodymind. There is a magical power to listening that bases itself in the human desire to be heard and to be understood. Interestingly, in its early days psychotherapy was referred to as "the listening cure."

Just so, we listen, we observe. Without further intervention, we allow the client to do with this fulcrum what they will.

Calmness of mind does not mean you should stop your activity.
Real calmness should be found in activity itself.
— Shunryu Suzuki

Monitor for Change

Monitoring for change — we are watchful for objective signs of a deeper bodymind experience.

While we hold the fulcrum, actively listening and observing, the client has an open space, a restful time in which to let go of any tensions that no longer serve them. Indeed, as we sustain the gesture or upon its end, it is common to notice an objective change in the client—what we term a "working sign."

How do we know how long to sustain a handshake? How do we know in life when it is the "right" moment to make—or break—contact? Usually there is a perceptible signal. In a handshake, it may be a breaking of eye contact, a release of pressure, a change in breathing, or even a smile that signals satisfactory greeting. At this point, were we to continue contact, the other person would pull their energy back and wait for us to release their hand.

Monitoring for change helps us apply the "Goldilocks principle" with regard to time. For a fulcrum to be fully effective it needs to be not too long, not too short, but just right. "Just right" comes about from paying close attention to the signs of bodymind change.

This sacred sensing of the most ideal measure for a sustained positive experience is something we consciously cultivate through Deep Massage. We endeavor to use just the right pressure, and with observed change as our guide, just the right timing.

The therapist need not wait for change. Monitoring is a commitment to observing, to listening. If the client doesn't visibly respond, we move on, trying to err of the side of the fulcrum being too short rather than too long. Better not to overstay a welcome.

Clearly Disengage

Clearly disengaging — we show trust in the client's inner wisdom by letting go.

There is the miracle of conscious meeting; there is also the fine art of consciously saying goodbye. When we perceive change, or, in some other manner, sense that the time for this fulcrum to end has come, it is important that we leave interface in a clear manner.

This means the disengagement is neither too abrupt nor too lingering. We exit in a way that gracefully moves back through the previous steps. The gesture ends, we let go of the slack we've taken up. Client and therapist have a moment in time to experience themselves as individuals with their own separate boundaries before another significant movement is made together.

Without the therapist's input, the client now has precious moments in which to integrate and assimilate the experience of this fulcrum. In most bodywork we learn "moves" with our hands. However, sometimes the client's most powerful experiences occur when he or she is not being massaged, moments in which to savor the experience of feeling, without pressure, an amplified, clearer energy flow and a renewed sense of structural harmony.

Imagine conversations you've had in which you felt you could not get a word in edgewise. Bodywork without significant pauses is like that—somewhat exhausting to the nervous system. Deep Massage, like music and other art forms, benefits from well-placed silences and open spaces. Clearly disengaging reminds us why religious custom considers the seventh day of creation as a most holy day of rest. Letting go is always the ultimate gesture of the creative process.

As a therapist your letting go gives living permission to the client to also let go of any physical or energetic problems they no longer wish to hold; to rest, and to begin the next of phase of their creative life.

Pausing

The meaning of "the power of the great" shows itself in the fact that one pauses.

— I Ching

Each of the above steps embodies what I call "palpatory courtesy." As we build the fulcrum, it is important that we pause at each step, however briefly, to acknowledge and respect each new psychophysical boundary encountered. Pause before contacting and center yourself. Take out the looseness; then pause before taking up the slack. Take up the slack; then pause to acknowledge clear contact with the client's tension. Then move in a curve or press into a point while "actively listening" for their response—this is a kind of pausing within our doing, manifesting, as Shunryu Suzuki says, "calmness in activity." When we sense it is time to let go, we disengage and pause before beginning the next fulcrum.

These pauses demonstrate we are attentive to the distinct layers of the person's sensory world. We are saying to their nervous system that now we are engaging their touch receptors, now their pressure receptors, now their proprioceptors. With this deep courtesy, the person feels safest to go deeply within, because we have fully respected their boundaries; we have demonstrated our trustworthiness through touch.

Much of the secret to cultivating the highest quality of touch lies in the care and respect conveyed by thoughtful pauses.

Communication is a two-way street. We call and they respond. Pausing allows time and space for the client's response. Every pause, even as brief as half a second, allows for an entirely different, deeper response in body, mind, and spirit.

Working Signs of Bodymind Healing

The thing that brings human value back to experience is the touching of it with human presence.

—Steve Gilligan

In his book, *Focusing*, psychotherapist Eugene Gendlin referred to a study that queried what differences there might be among individuals who experienced positive change as a result of psychotherapy and individuals who did not. The answer was that those who made the most progress in therapy experienced a tangible, bodily felt change.

Throughout life we often access our sense of truth more deeply and directly through the body than through the mind. Knowing things in your gut, sensing what is true in your heart, feeling grounded in what you stand for—these are just some of the ways in which bodily-felt experience manifests the deepest kind of knowing.

Deep Massage recognizes that we are practicing a sensory and motor skill, an art and science that require observation as much as action. In a full life and in this work, what we sense is as important as what we do. We are looking, like bodymind detectives, for signs of greater health. It is said that the mammalian brain is specialized to read the emotions of other animals. Movement therapist Moshe Feldenkrais noted that in humans this capacity is so well developed as to represent an entirely new neurological capability.

In Deep Massage we call the movement toward greater health—the positive state of internal shift, re-arrangement, re-orientation, change—the working state. The signs of this working state that we can perceive we call the working signs. Working signs are largely objective signs of the healing trajectory of the bodymind during therapy sessions.

Between waking and dreaming,
there is a third thing – guess it.

– Antonio Machado

Both consciously and unconsciously, clients do inner work to become healthier. It is natural to want to feel better, to seek greater enjoyment in life, to be happier. This is the momentum every therapist rides upon.

Of course, every client also experiences frustration in his or her life and inner work. Often this is the result of difficult upbringings that leave unresolved issues in us from childhood that can hold us back from fulfilling ourselves as adults. Sometimes physical injuries leave tensions that bind up our energy and structure. Sometimes narrow-mindedness or educational shortcomings can leave a person without the tools most needed for achieving self-fulfillment.

Whatever the reason, Deep Massage brings essential information to the bodymind, which facilitates the inner work of the client. Enlightened touch will facilitate the unbinding of body, mind, and spirit.

Deep Massage — enlightened touch — depends as much on our eyes as on our hands. What do you do with your eyes when you do bodywork? In Deep Massage, as soon as you are confident that your body and hands are clearly placed for a given fulcrum, allow your eyes to play over the whole person.

We touch locally, yet we observe globally. Watch the eyes of the client, their breathing, and the other signs described below.

Deep seeing is really understanding. We need to work with understanding as well as with our hands. People want to be seen. Notice how the beneficent gaze of an approving parent lets the child feel both energized and safe in their life. So it is for our clients. They feel the kindness of our observation skills and let go more deeply as a result of our attention.

What are the signs that we have successfully touched a client in such a way that they are bringing human value to neglected or new facets of themselves? What are the working signs of bodymind healing?

The Eyes

Each day we gage people through the eyes—the "windows to the soul." Deep Massage therapists commonly look at changes in the eyes for manifestations of inner changes during the session. Working signs here may include:

• Eyes suddenly opening as if a bright idea has just occurred.

• Eyes suddenly closing, conveying the feeling that the client has just gone deeper inside themselves.

• Rapid eye movements with the eyelids fluttering like butterfly wings, indicating the client is hovering in a fertile state between sleeping and waking.

Rapid movement of the eyes beneath the lids, while intriguing, is not considered a working sign; it is a sign that the client is asleep and dreaming. An assumption here is that healing more likely occurs with the mutual engagement of both the conscious and unconscious. Healing has more to do with deeply awakening than with going to sleep.

Facial Expression

The eyes contribute significantly to overall facial expression—a form of nonverbal communication under the control of muscles that are unique in the whole body. Whereas most muscles attach to bones, the facial muscles attach to one another. Facial muscles pull on other facial muscles, their associated connective tissues, and the skin under which they lie. This gives rise to an incredible plasticity and infinite variation of facial expression.

By the time we are adults, we have all seen countless faces. We receive, almost instantaneously, deep and distinct impressions from every face we see. It is difficult to put into words what you learn from someone's face because we "see" people mostly with deeper parts of ourselves. Yet it offers such a generous revelation of inner worlds!

In faces you can detect chronic shock, compassion, inclinations to anger, long-held grief, thoughtfulness, love, mirth, affection, phoniness, joy—the list of emotions and their combinations is endless. You may see a healthy glow or the pallor of depletion. In the disappearance of "worry lines" or the release of jaw tension you may see the qualitative shifts toward more relaxed states.

When you do therapy, keep your attention primarily at interface when you are touching. Yet secondarily observe for working signs throughout the body, including the face. Have faith that your years of looking at faces will guide you to touch in a manner more responsive to the unique nature of the client and the moment in which he or she is working. The amount of pressure, the timing for a stroke, the quality of emotion that you respond with and embody in your touch—these all may be beautifully informed by what is evidenced in the face.

It may help at times to put what you are feeling and seeing into words in your mind. In this way you also ideally mobilize your logical and imaginative mind to contribute as needed.

For news of the heart, ask the face.

— Cambodian proverb

The Breath

*Breath is the bridge
between matter and spirit.*

If the eyes are the windows to the soul, then breath is surely the window to the spirit. Indeed, spirit resides just there between "in-spire" and "re-spire." You take over 17,000 breaths every day. As an example, multiply that times twenty-five years and you have hundreds of millions of breaths. You are experienced in breathing!

Each time we watch the breathing of our clients, we observe from a vantage point of vast experience. We intuitively recognize breaths of deep relaxation, anxiety, held-in pride, personal deflation, grief, laughing breaths, sighs of relief, of despair, breaths of serenity, sleep, or excitement.

As with facial expression, note that through this working sign you are able to some extent to track the trajectory of the client's energy. Like a shooting star, you aren't seeing energy's source directly; you can't tell when it started or even where it exactly is. But like that shooting star, it is real, and seeing the breath provides a real window into that spirit's journey in time and space.

Let your gaze, your touch, your breath, and your mind meet their journeying spirit,

body, and breath with deeper responsiveness thanks to this fascinating working sign.

In Deep Massage and Zero Balancing, one particular trajectory that can help you connect more deeply with the client is to respect what we call "the working breath cycle." This is graphed by a series of gentle up and down curves, signifying regular breath rhythms, followed by lesser curves or a straight line, signifying shallower breaths, or an apnea, a temporary cessation of breath. This is followed in turn by a larger breath than normal—a "hyperpnea"—and then the resumption of a normal breathing rhythm.

This working breath cycle is a dependable sign of energetic/neurologic completion. In everyday life these often occur at the end of something we've been doing when we take a break or when we complete it.

The working breath cycle gives us a very clear sign that enhances our connection, whereby we coordinate our fulcrum timing with the rhythms of the client's inner work.

Voice Vitality

Attunement to voice almost instantaneously allows us to recognize who someone is, in part through the timbre, rhythm, volume, and melodies of vocal expression. There are two contexts in massage when the voice tells us much of what we need to know: during the pre-session interview and periodically during the therapy itself.

Before an initial session I always take an extensive life/health history. I want the relevant facts. During this time I am also consciously listening not only to what they say but how they say it.

As with facial expression, the impressions from the voice go first to my unconscious. If you ask yourself, "What is this voice telling me?" you will find the words of your own inner voice detecting deeply important things about this person:

- The tempo of their mind
- The flatness or variability of their emotional state
- Their sincerity or relative lack thereof
- Their word choice and grammar, suggestive of their educational experience
- Their self-awareness
- Their energy level

During a session, I am particularly interested in receiving, at least once or twice, verbal feedback about the client's experience. I usually ask, "How are you doing?" and listen carefully to the response.

Among those things that indicate we are on the right track:

- A relatively quick or positive response
- A vitality in the voice that suggests the client is experiencing a net energy gain
- A clear and strong choice of words
- A vocal tone that matches the words

Conversely, if the response is markedly delayed; if the voice sounds weak or far away; if the words are not clear; or if the client's words and tone don't match, I take that as an indication to course-correct.

Be particularly sensitive and aware, as these may be signs of depletion. When I suspect a net loss of energy or a lack of healthy connection, I will adjust my touch, frequently making it clearer, more up-tempo. I may try establishing a stronger interface and make sure to verbally check in with the client again after a few minutes to assure the course correction has been effective.

Body Tissue Change

Hands flow, tension goes.
And now is the time
for the soft way of being.

— Elliot Greene

With high-quality touch, a common working sign is a qualitative change. A hard place will rather suddenly soften. A cold place will warm up. A place that felt unalive will feel like someone's turned on the water and it is flowing through.

Movement

Small movements, called *kriyas* from the Sanskrit meaning of "purified action" — are involuntary movements of a body part, such as slight movements of a finger or the hand, the feet or a leg.

This is like a twitch, seen often when a client "falls" asleep. It relates to the working state as it indicates the client has just dropped into the unconscious and then rebounded. Do make sure that the client isn't just asleep. Commonly if you ask the client, they will say they were aware of having made the movement but that it wasn't something consciously done. At times, the client's whole body may visibly and spontaneously re-arrange itself during a session and come to rest in a more relaxed, aligned posture on the table.

Borborygmus or Swallowing

The letting go of tension manifests neurologically as a shift in the autonomic nervous system. The shift is from the stress response, the sympathetic side, to the parasympathetic side, the relaxation and repose response. Overall this causes a global change in our circulatory patterns. Under stress, circulation shifts from our internal organs to the voluntary and cardiac muscles so that we may take fast and decisive action if necessary.

In a state of repose, by contrast, circulation is re-directed to our center and to the re-building, nourishing functions of our visceral organs. This enhances actions related to digestion, assimilation, and elimination. Thus, we may see the working sign of swallowing, a sign of increased salivation that accompanies the parasympathetic side. We will commonly hear sounds of increased intestinal movement, or "borborygmus."

Sometimes clients will apologize for bowel rumblings during a session. I am happy to assure them that it's a good sign!

Client Reports

Many times, though I won't sense anything in particular, the client will report an unusual and positive experience. These can vary widely. Some reports of working signs may include seeing vibrant colors with the eyes closed; experiencing an emotional release; recalling a vivid memory; feeling a definite beneficial change in body sensation, body image or mood; or having a sudden insight or a lifting of confusion.

Serenity

Sometimes the atmosphere in the room just seems to change. I may think, *"Someone has turned off the air-conditioning,"* then I realize that it's actually the vibration in the room that has shifted. This is a bit trickier than the other working signs as it is less objectively obvious. But do note when the therapy room seems qualitatively more serene. You will certainly know you are on the right track if the client confirms your sensibility.

Synchronicity

Synchronicity is not necessarily generated by the session itself. Synchronous happenings can precipitate a deeper experience, whether or not they are caused by our work—for instance, the sudden parting of clouds and a sunbeam warming the face of the client, or the sound of a child's carefree laughter, or a birdsong at the perfect moment. Whether through happenstance or through spontaneously entwined destinies, positive synchronicities enhance the session by making the client feel an even deeper sense of delight.

The universe became the accomplice of all my wishes.

— Jacques Lusseyran

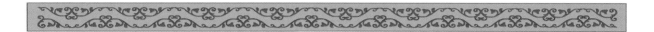

Part Two

Practical Tips and Basic Techniques

Touch affects the physical body and more. It affects us three-dimensionally and in yet deeper ways. Touch communicates with the energy running through us, illumining our hearts, minds, and spirit.

How does touch, as with poetic verse, achieve this transformative power? Touch has seven dimensions through which we glean insight and facilitate healing. Each dimension enhances our appreciation for the profound potential in every relationship offered us by deep touch. These seven dimensions are: Contact, Movement, Breath, Graceful Verticality, Heart, Understanding, and Alchemy.

Here we will present chapters that offer instruction in the basic Deep Massage techniques, alternating with lucid discussions, drawn from a new philosophy of touch, that explore the Seven Dimensions of Touch which enliven the art and science of our profession.

You will learn in these chapters a series of wonderful fulcrums for the back, shoulders and arms, pelvis, posterior and anterior thighs, lower legs, front torso, neck, and head. Once grounded in practical context, we can see how the whole person manifests uniquely in the anatomy and energetics of that part of their body.

The goal, practically speaking, is that you will become skillful with Deep Massage. The first step is to learn and practice in a logical sequence the fulcrums described and illustrated in this book.

Basic Deep Massage Protocol

Fists Down the Erectors

Nine Points

Ironing up the Erectors

Levator Scapula

Posterior Neck – Trapezius, Semispinalis, Multifidus/Rotatores

Gluteus Maximus

Hamstrings

Gastrocnemius/Soleus

Tensor Fascia Lata, Gluteus Medius, and Gluteus Minimus

Iliotibial Band

Rectus Femoris

Peroneus Longus (aka Fibularis)

Tibialis Anterior

Half-Moon Vector through the Legs

Rectus Abdominis

Pectoralis Major

Biceps Brachii

Triceps Brachii

Trapezius (supine)

Scalenes

Facial Muscles

Epicranius

Half-Moon Vector through the Neck

Half-Moon Vector through the Legs

The rest of this chapter offers some basic information that is primarily useful for non-professionals or beginning students. If you are a professional massage therapist, feel free to skim the familiar material, but do pay close attention to some of the suggestions below, which are particular to Deep Massage and will prove helpful as reminders or as additions to your practice.

Supplies

Massage Table

Massage, like music or writing, is blissfully basic in terms of the supplies required. At the time I bought my first massage table, most were handmade or made by very small manufacturers. I remember, having bought it, carrying it down the stairs of a Chicago apartment building, filled with a welling sense of joy and anticipation. Perhaps something inside me knew this was an instrument of destiny, as the guitar had been for my previous thirty years.

All major table manufacturers make excellent products now. If you don't already have one, feel confident to buy one, either online (after thorough research) or, preferably, from a local massage supply store or massage school where you can see and try out the actual table. I generally recommend a table-width of 29" for a shorter person; 30" is probably most common.

The table height should be adjustable. Here is how to find the appropriate table height for Deep Massage. Stand up and extend your arm downwards, with the wrists bent back so your hands would lie palms down on the table. For Deep Massage the table should be approximately 2" lower than where your extended palm would be. For a larger client you may consider setting the table height even lower.

The point of table height with Deep Massage is that as much as possible, it is preferable to lean in to your work, letting gravity be the therapist, rather than pressing in with bodily effort. Although at times effort is unavoidable, please refrain from unnecessary effort! I say if you could use the gravitational field of an entire planet or your own force, which would you choose?

Draping

Try to use sheets that are pleasant to the skin, such as a flannel or a smooth, high-quality cotton. For the sake of warmth and clear boundaries, be mindful to only uncover the area of the body on which you are working.

Lubricant

In Deep Massage we do not use lubricant unless absolutely necessary. Just as with force, the lubricant you need is naturally already there. Your skin and that of your client have naturally produced oils (sebum) and moisture (perspiration) on the surface. Swedish massage uses lubricant because its primary focus is on repeated flowing strokes that stimulate circulation and relaxation. Artificial lubricants help us glide over the surface.

Deep Massage focuses on contacting the client deeply, facilitating changes in the muscles and connective tissues and more clearly connecting to the nervous system and energy as well as structure. In Deep Massage, we prefer that nothing blur the interface; our goal is to sink in and stimulate deeper bodymind movement.

There are exceptions. Some clients may have copious body hair, making them sensitive to the pulling sensation from massage. Some may have very dry skin, or express a strong preference for lubricant. In such cases I recommend using cream rather than oil and even then only the minimum necessary to make the client feel comfortable.

If you plan to combine Swedish massage with Deep Massage, I recommend using only the minimum necessary amount of lubricant for doing the Swedish strokes first, allowing the lubricant to sink in (again, cream is better than oil for this), then follow that with Deep Massage. This honors the client's boundaries, focusing initially on superficial work before working into deeper structural and energetic layers.

Bolsters and Pillows

Support for the full array of body types is facilitated by having pillows or bolsters, which you can get from a massage school, massage supply store, or online. Most commonly, these will be placed under the ankles when the client is prone or, in the supine position, under the knees, to help the client feel more comfort in the lower back.

In Deep Massage it also is useful to have a smaller, less thick pillow that can be positioned under the client's head. Use this only for clients whose chins, when they lie face up, are higher up than their foreheads. For those clients, the little pillow will help restore a healthier alignment through the whole spine.

The Therapist's Body Mechanics/Comfort

Ideally, massage is a healing activity for both giver and receiver. With that in mind, settle into an optimal psychophysical tone before you put your hands on your client. Tune your instrument!

Keep your legs spread at about shoulder width. Feel grounded, well aligned and buoyant through your skeletal system. Breathe freely through your body, allowing your shoulders to rise and fall gently as you breathe in and out. Feel a sense of openness in your shoulder joint between the shoulder blades, chest, and the upper arm. Imagine a "cushion" of air between your arms and your torso. Let your body overall be slightly rounded and soft, yet feel your strength as well as your gracefulness. Enjoy feeling grounded and buoyant. A therapist at work should look like a skilled martial artist doing tai chi, relaxed while nonetheless effectively mobilizing one's energy in the movement.

While you work, relax your hands as much as possible. The body is mostly water. As you explore the client's body, if you find a hard place, remember it is mostly water, therefore you can sink or melt into it—you don't need or want to push your way through. When your mind and hands truly know this, you will maintain only as much fixity of the hands as is necessary to provide a clear contact. Generally let your fingers be at a natural distance from one another, not pulled together or spread forcefully apart.

Exercise

If you find your arms, hands, or any body part easily fatiguing, consider modifying your exercise routine. Some people's hands and wrists may need more length, others more strength. There is an excellent book, *Save Your Hands*, with explanations and exercises for hand care. If you are just beginning massage, try alternating two-minute immersions of your hands and arms in icy then hot water up to the elbow.

Most skillful therapists combine overall lengthening exercises with strengthening

ones. Yoga, weight training, and aerobic exercise are all ideal. Some activities combine these forms—e.g., martial arts. I encourage you to do the exercise forms that you enjoy the most, then consider if there is something missing and how you might most enjoyably add it. For instance, people drawn to yoga may need to balance it with more aerobic exercise, yet prefer intoxicating outdoor workouts to repetitive work in the gym.

Client's arm and hand placement

Generally, in Deep Massage, if the client is supine, we recommend the client's hands rest on his or her belly. We want the client to experience a heightened energy flow. For this to happen, it is helpful to have the experience contained, so there is a net energy gain, rather than it just spilling out or over.

One way to accomplish this is simply to have the client rest his/her hands on the belly or possibly the lower chest, depending on their anatomy. We all recognize the comfortable feeling of containment, sitting sometimes with our arms or legs crossed. Similarly, in Zen meditation, individuals sit in a cross-legged position with their hands in front of the lower belly. In this manner as well, Deep Massage is a two-person meditation, the client in the meditating role and the therapist facilitating.

Direction of strokes

A primary purpose of Swedish massage is to enhance circulation. Therefore, Swedish strokes are generally directed toward the heart. In Deep Massage the focus is on lengthening and freeing the muscles, fascia, bones, and joints, as well as freeing the flow of energy through the bodymind. The stroke/fulcrum directions, especially in the extremities, are toward their distal ends—toward the hands, feet, or head. Anatomically speaking, then, we work on lengthening, primarily from origin to insertion.

Work the less affected side first

If the client's complaint is, for instance, the right shoulder, I will tend to address the left shoulder first. In this way, when you get to the right shoulder, the client will already be more relaxed. Additionally the nervous system correlates tension and release across the body. Working the less affected side first will already open up the more problematic area.

Training

When I first started my studies, there were fewer than 50 massage schools in the U.S., and much training was apprenticeship-based. Now massage therapy has become a viable, mainstream occupation. There are hundreds of schools, and as in most fields, some good, many adequate, some poor.

Massage school can and should rank amongst the best and most revolutionary experiences of one's life. Learning anatomy and physiology, how to move and breathe, how to start your own business, how to relate healthily to other people, how to provide relief of muscle tension and injury, how to touch so that stress is deeply relieved—these skills will serve you in many ways for the rest of your life. Often, near the beginning of each class, I am filled with excitement and think, *Everyone should know this!*

If you have not yet considered going to massage school, I hope this book encourages you to do so. It is still a relatively inexpensive form of higher education. Research your options thoroughly. Do not make a decision based on one person's opinion or a few online reviews. Find and interview at least five therapists in your area, talk with employers, and do look extensively online. Is their website a good source of information?

Visit the school and bring questions. Look at their educational handouts and their facilities and see if you can sit in for at least 15 minutes of an ongoing class.

If you are therapist, you obviously have an appetite for more. I encourage you to continue your studies in Deep Massage and other advanced forms of massage and bodywork.

I hope—and this book is a manifestation of this hope—that the things we learn from good massage training are eventually integrated into mainstream elementary and secondary school curricula. How to touch with respect and kindness, how one's body works, gracefulness, centering—this knowledge forms the basis for a healthier, saner, happier world.

Integrating Other Modalities within Deep Massage

Ultimately, in the widest sense, Deep Massage is what enables you to affect the client most profoundly in a positive way. Deep Massage is certainly not limited to the techniques described in this book—these constitute merely the basic protocols. There are advanced Deep Massage techniques not included here, and there are many other modalities that can affect someone deeply.

The primary question to ask is: which modality best serves the client? Secondarily, which modalities do you most enjoy using? Just as an artist may prefer a certain medium, therapists often do their best work working with the modalities they find most compelling.

How may other modalities be usefully integrated within Deep Massage? There are two primary goals to consider. One is to respect boundaries; the other is to amplify integration.

Before doing a Deep Massage fulcrum, it is useful to become familiar with the area where you will be working. This may involve a brief effleurage/gliding stroke or kneading. If you avoid plunging into deeper territory unannounced, it shows a respect for boundaries. It also gives you, and in a nonverbal sense, your client, more kinesthetic information about tensions or freedom in the area to be addressed.

To amplify the experience of integration consider as well gently rocking the whole body or limb after a fulcrum; doing one or more gliding strokes over the whole area; giving a gentle pat or briefly resting your hands on the body. These are artful integrations for you to add based on your intuition regarding what may result in the client feeling most complete and cared for.

With these integrative movements, the client will more assuredly experience not just the effective release of their various parts, but also a more caring and integrated whole-body experience. I recommend that you indeed include these introductory and integrative movements in your Deep Massage from the start.

Later on, when you truly feel fluent with Deep Massage, there are other possible combinations. Each combination requires that you have enough fluency with Deep Massage to impart a complete experience in as little as half an hour. I recommend including no more than fifteen minutes of these additional modalities:

- Preceding Deep Massage with some Swedish massage.
- Following Deep Massage with other integrative modalities such as craniosacral work or Zero Balancing.
- Following a short Deep Massage with a short pure energy work such as Jin Shin Do.

What to avoid? *Above all, do not overwork the client.* Do not go too deep or take overly long. If you are integrating other modalities, it is generally advisable to complete the entire session in less than one hour.

When you are engaging both structure and energy, time is experienced differently. It is a more intense engagement. A full hour session is usually more than enough time for the client to experience the benefits— any longer and you risk the client feeling overworked or depleted. Less is more!

The steps in the Deep Massage Basic Protocol are described in the chapters that follow. In Chapter 19, Session Design, you will find more details on how they may be combined and ways to integrate them with other massage and bodywork modalities you may practice.

Important Reminder on Applying Pressure

Even though I emphasize sensitivity when I am teaching, I find that students, when they hear "Deep Massage" often assume that this means "Press Harder."

Please be explicitly reminded that this is not the case.

Deep Massage is an approach quite distinct from "Deep Tissue" massage. In Deep Massage we use only enough pressure for the client to feel well-met. We do not accomplish tension release primarily through applying pressure.

When appropriately met at interface, the client is able to let go from inside out and effect the release of tension and realize a deeper experience of health.

Please remember: if you are inclined to add more pressure to make sure you are being effective, please don't. Have faith in your client's ability to release.

Contact—The First Dimension of Touch

It is not the educational intention,
rather it is the meeting which is educationally fruitful.

— Martin Buber

The Myth of Modalities

There is a mythos about the field of massage and bodywork. The belief is that modalities are all-powerful and vast and that practitioners should be consumers of these modalities if they want to be supremely successful therapists. In the market culture, the product or service to be consumed is given more importance than the individual who will consume it.

This turns the truth on its head. In bodywork it is the individuals—the therapist and client—who are the source of healing. The modality is of secondary importance. Nonetheless, most massage bodywork training consists of modality training.

Let us waken from the spell of believing that modalities heal people—that craniosacral work is powerful, Reiki sublime, Rolfing fantastic. Not true. Modalities have zero power. The true healing power of bodywork is wielded by the person who is giving it and the client who is receiving it. Healing is done by the client with help from the therapist.

Modalities are tools at best, brainwashing at worst. As Andrew Taylor Still stated, "The body contains all the healing substances it needs." Every therapist with decent training and the simplest desire to help others by touching them has all the healing energy—

ideas, feelings, movements—he or she needs to help. A truly caring individual has more power than all modalities combined. If I have the choice of an advanced practitioner who is full of himself, or a basic practitioner who genuinely cares, I will go for the care every time.

If love is present, we open up, and if it's not, we don't. Perhaps love is that which opens. I may not be able to teach a student to love. I can't require it for their grades. But that doesn't make it any less primary in what we are trying to accomplish. It is harder to educate the character, the person of the therapist, on who to be in the therapeutic relationship than to come right out and tell them what to do.

Deep caring remains our first concern and chief resource, with technique running a distant second. How can we rigorously develop the skill to love? How can we be rigorous in the study of this incredible primary content of our work?

First and foremost, realize the primary role of deep care in massage. It is the reason why people are attracted to this profession. Tragically, some schools and workshop marketers are consistently selling off this precious truth for the falsity of modality instruction.

Our source and destination must continue to be the ever mysterious and wondrous LIFE and LOVE. To break the spell of modality worship, the best tool I have come up with is a better understanding of the seven dimensions inherent in touch.

Contact—The First Dimension of Touch

Over the years I've received massage therapy work from many students and colleagues. From this receiving perspective I have observed seven specific dimensions of touch that compose structurally and energetically effective work, regardless of modality. The literally multi-dimensional experience of touch is the foundation that existentially precedes and underlies all bodywork modalities.

The first dimension of touch occurs when we lay our hands upon someone. Just laying down a hand establishes a point or area of contact. Remember from geometry, a point has one dimension. In this rigorous, geometric sense, the first level of touch is one dimensional, the laying on of a hand, establishing a point of contact. Yet how powerful this is!

This single dimension of basic contact sums up everything eloquently depicted in Michelangelo's famous Sistine Chapel painting, where God and Adam reach toward each other. The power of this picture is that it depicts with stunning visual beauty the creation of life.

Creation occurs in the moment and in the space of touching another. This is the relationship. Two people sharing their energies through touch create an additional force. How can we honor and further empower this incredible opportunity?

First of all, we sense and accept its reality. When two conscious beings touch, it creates a structural occurrence. Energetically, however, it is a miracle. The combined vibration of these two beings—what Martin Buber called the "I-Thou relationship"—commences. This is the incredible power inherent in the first dimension of touch.

There are two aspects to this dimension. The first has to do with location. Where do we decide to initiate contact and why? If where we first make contact becomes habitual and not the result of a sacred decision, then we've squandered an incredible opportunity.

To make this decision we need the knowledge of anatomy, especially musculoskeletal. Often we can tell if a therapist is competent simply by where they first place their hands. Knowledge of each individual's appropriate boundaries is also necessary. In one person the face might be the best place to start, in another, it might be the last. As you refine your intuitive knowledge of an individual's needs, you can most appropriately choose the optimal starting place.

The energetic aspect of the first dimension of touch has to do with conscious and intuitive decisions regarding how we touch the client. Do we use a lot of pressure or none at all? Do we bring a lot of energy into our hands or a modest amount? Do we touch with firmness, love, consolation, authority, curiosity? The vastness of meanings conveyed by touch is daunting. Let us inhabit this vastness, enjoy the majestic, mysterious aspect of keeping open the question: How shall we meet?

Psycho—mechanics and the Organization of Awareness

Since energy follows awareness, refining the energetic aspect of basic contact involves the organization of awareness. For the first dimension, then, the question is not just where and how do you place your hand, but equally where do you place your consciousness?

Ida Rolf, a genius of modern bodywork, spoke of many bodies as being "randomly" organized. Pointing out that children, for example, learn to walk by hook or by crook, stumbling awkwardly across a room in search of the nearest graspable structure, Ida Rolf underscored the almost totally unmet need for movement education in our society.

In massage school we attempt to address this need through the teaching of biomechanics, in which efficiency of posture and breath are emphasized. Accompanying biomechanics training is the specific choreography of hand and body movements particular to the specific modality the student is learning. (How beautiful a choreography it can be!)

In our society and in our massage schools there is a yet deeper choreography for our focus. This is the equally important choreography of awareness. In our regular schooling we are not taught directly how to think or how to access with alertness and curiosity the awareness of our own thoughts, movements, or feelings. As with the largely non-existent movement education, students are left to structure their awareness of themselves and the world around them without systematic guidance. As a result, most of us grow up not just with "random" bodies, but also with "random" minds. Particularly when under stress, people often are strictly reactive, on autopilot, displaying the level of psychic organization of the average pinball machine.

What then are the steps toward an appropriate choreography of awareness, a *psycho-mechanics* to parallel the biomechanics of massage?

A primary goal is to literally and figuratively pay attention to the "matter at hand." Earlier I described this focused state as "interface." Remember, working at interface involves the energy and structure of the therapist meeting with the energy and structure of the client. Generally, this meeting takes place where our hands, elbows, or other contacting part touches the body of the client. It may also be, as in the case of a stretch, where our force has the most impact. For instance, in a hamstring stretch, although we may not be touching the hamstrings directly, our structural and energetic impact will be experienced there.

Even more than intention, interface is a direct way of focusing during a massage, since intention implies a cerebral directive. With interface, your attention is literally centered on the place and the moment where the two of you—client and therapist—bodily and consciously meet. The act of centering on interface itself involves a radical organizing of consciousness. Until we've centered on something, there is no point of reference around which our consciousness is organized.

Without centering, we are like a body without gravity, adrift with no reference point for up, down, forward, or back. With a center, a homing for our awareness, we can become conscious of when we are focused and when we're not. As in meditation, in which the awareness may be centered on the breath, the tip of the nose, or the area just below the navel, healthy psycho-mechanics in bodywork involves being centered on the place—the interface—where our structures and energies meet.

However, as in meditation, it is not the goal, nor is it truly possible, to remain unalterably centered at interface. Your awareness may wander—at times to your movements, at others to your emotions, your thoughts, or your sensations. Your job as a therapist is basically to keep bringing your awareness back "home," to center.

The role of home is not as a place we always stay, but as a place to which we return. Frequently, during a session, we bring our wandering awareness back to interface. Then our clients experience our commitment to be truly present with them, not just in body but in mind and spirit as well.

The psycho-mechanics of bodywork differ from meditation in this crucial respect: part of therapy involves conscious problem-solving. The wandering of our awareness is more relevant and, at times, necessary. We need to be ready to access all of ourselves to be fully present. In the words of the French essayist, Jacques Riviere, "The sincere man stops at each level of himself and chooses what he needs to form his truth."

For instance, I may be doing shoulder work and staying mostly at interface when I have the insight that the pain the client described in their history may be more appropriately relieved through specific work on the supraspinatus than the general trapezius work I had planned. I then access my anatomical "data banks," visualizing the precise origin, route, and angle of the supraspinatus. I deepen my focus, as quickly and gracefully as possible, with interface at the place that is called for, and work there with heightened clarity and relevance.

Similarly, I may bring awareness to my emotions when during a session I might feel, for example, anger. Does this anger relate to an event I experienced earlier in the day or am I "picking up" on the held-in anger of my client? If so, what might be the appropriate content of my touch? Once I've sorted that out, I come back to interface and hopefully to a deepened, clearer emotional communication between myself and the client.

During a session, I may also notice unnecessary tension creeping into my body or my breathing. People pick up not just on what we preach with our hands, but, perhaps more so, on what we practice with our whole bodies. It is vastly important to set a psychophysical example for one's client. Trying, for instance, to relieve shoulder pain without freedom in my own shoulders is therapeutically hypocritical. I bring my awareness to my tension, let it go, breathing, moving back now a freer person and more gracefully interfacing.

There is an elegant integrity when we model in our body and being what we hope for our clients. That way as they get healthier, so do we.

Finally, during a session I may fall into the mistaken frame of reference that I am performing therapy on a passive client; that it's all up to me. In this case, I've created what Buber would call an "I-it" relationship. To restore the "I-Thou," I access my spiritual sense, the knowledge that we are equal and in a deep way connected in this world. I bring this acknowledged kinship-with-all-life feeling back to our interface. I also trust that it is the client's wisdom, not my own, that determines the extent to which letting go will serve them.

This is the dance of therapy, the delicate ballet of awareness in which we inhabit mostly interface, while circulating in appropriate ways through our mind, emotions, body, and spirit. This is the psycho-mechanics of bodywork.

Experiencing a New Wholeness

Therapy begins with basic contact, the first dimension. In this dimension, where we touch, how we touch, and how we organize our awareness combine to create the therapeutic effect.

The belief that modalities are the source of our power, as in "I hear that craniosacral work is really good" or "What does Trigger Point work do?" is a widespread fallacy. In our market economy, many people try to sell you their product and convince you that you need it. The underlying social belief is this: the only thing worth having is what you don't yet have. The truth is quite the opposite. We already have everything we need. To revisit the words of Andrew Taylor Still, osteopathy's illustrious founder, it is as true for the therapist as for the client that "the body contains all the healing substances it needs." When one caring person touches another, healing—the experience of a new wholeness—takes place. Healing is in the nature of people coming together.

We don't need modalities, we need each other. The power lies in each one of us. Let us organize our awareness and touch and enjoy this incredible capacity to really meet one another. Touching with an appropriately organized body, mind, emotions, and spirit, is fruitful. It is creative. It is an honor to be in a profession where truly meeting another person is the entire point.

The Back: Anatomy, Energy, and Fulcrums

There Is No Back

Strictly speaking, there is no back. No more is there a "back" of the body than we would talk about the back of an orange or a banana. The human torso is a slightly flattened cylinder with the spine running right through our center.

Though we can feel the so-called "backbones," these are just the little bony tails, the tips of the spinous processes, projecting posteriorly from the vertebral bodies. The main structural, weight-bearing elements of the spine are the vertebral bodies that lie closer toward our center.

I remember years ago in Chicago I had a lawyer client who appreciated my excitement for learning anatomy and offered to arrange a tour of the Cook County morgue.

One day we headed on down, and it felt like *down*, to the underworld of the morgue. I saw cadavers of those recently deceased, some of whom had been reported on the previous night's TV news. They still appeared vital, as if they could jump up at any second and say hello.

I looked at the body of one young man who'd recently passed. Where it seemed his stomach ordinarily would be located there was a reddish column. At first I had no idea what it was, but soon realized it was the front of his vertebral column! It appeared that his spine was closer to the front of his body than to the back. Since then I've never forgotten that the spine is as much in our center as it is posterior in our bodies.

Anatomy

Skeletally, the back consists of the vertebrae and the ribs. The back follows the course of the spine in the center to well down between the ilia, the two halves of the pelvis. If you were to draw a line between the two iliac crests, it would usually pass through the fourth lumbar vertebra. Beneath that level there is one more lumbar vertebra, the five fused vertebrae that constitute the sacrum and the five fused vertebrae forming the coccyx.

In its upper region, the back doesn't end at the top of the ribcage but extends up through the seven cervical vertebrae to the occipital bone at the base of the head. So "the back" is considerably longer than we generally envision it.

Muscularly the back is composed of a number of major layers.

The first is latissimus dorsi and the trapezius. Basically these amount to shoulder girdle muscles, the latissimus inserting on the front of the humerus and the trapezius inserting on the clavicle and scapula.

The next layer, the rhomboids, are also shoulder girdle muscles, inserting on the scapulae.

The third main muscle layer is the erector spinae, the first layer of back muscles proper. The erector spinae consist of three strands of muscle on either side of the spine. These three muscles climb up the back like vines climbing up a trellis. Laterally you have the iliocostalis attaching to the pelvis and ribs; intermediately, the longissimus, attaching to the pelvis, ribs, and vertebral transverse processes; and medially, just next to the spinous processes, the spinalis.

The fourth main layer is composed of the multifidus and rotatores running from the transverse processes up to the spinous processes.

The deepest layer is the quadratus lumborum, running from the "inner lip" of the iliac crest up to the transverse processes of the lumbar vertebrae and the undersurface of the 12th rib.

Structural Considerations

Over time, stress and the pull of gravity tend to result in a more compressed spine. Many of us spend too much of our time leaning forward rather than laying back; consequently our back muscles stay tense, and the spine compresses due to chronic muscle tension. Eventually that can lead to back pain, even to slipped discs, sprained ligaments, and strained muscles. The most important thing you can do for a back is to decompress it—to pull the muscles "back," taking the unneeded compression out from the spine—and to bring the back tissues back and down, so that the spine is better aligned and appropriately balanced in relation to the pelvis.

Energetics

Energetically the back carries the potential for many levels of existential meaning. Hippocrates himself said tellingly, "Get thee knowledge of the spine, for it is the source of many diseases." Equally it is the source of many virtues.

From the back, we acquire self-support, especially through the lumbar region. This can translate into the feeling of supporting oneself emotionally and/or economically. Many years back I learned I was going to be audited by the IRS. My back immediately went into spasm. I thought, "Ahh, this is absolutely textbook! Challenged support equals back spasm!"

Other possible energetic issues are often woven into the wisdom of everyday expressions. "Show some backbone!" recognizes the back as a primary source of strength and steadfastness. We've all heard the expression, "He's a spineless coward!" Courage is essential to a healthy back. The tonus of the back and abdominal muscles, in turn, helps sustain courage!

"Don't get your back up!" implying don't get angry, usually relates to the mid- and upper back and trapezius (think of an angry cat).

The thoracic spine area relates more to the realm of the heart. Chronic kyphosis or mid-scapular pain may relate to emotional issues such as holding back or holding in one's feelings, not speaking from the heart, or being overly guarded of one's heart.

Wilhelm Reich, the father of body-centered psychotherapy, said all neurosis manifests as a restriction of breath. The health of the thorax is fundamentally linked to the fullness of breath. Almost all thoracic back pain can thus be seen as a restriction of breath, and related emotional tension.

Fists Down the Erectors

At the beginning of a session you will most likely repeat this fulcrum three times—first once over lightly with medium speed, then in successive passes going just a bit slower and deeper.

Center yourself before putting your hands on the client. Stand at the head of the table in a comfortable position, your breathing relaxed and gently yet clearly focused. With the client lying face down (ideally with the head in a face cradle), place your loose fists, finger pads against your palms, at the top of the ribcage in the belly of the trapezius muscle.

Take out the looseness, making good contact. Before you begin the sliding motion down the back, take up the slack by stretching the tissue inferiorly. The initial inferior-ward traction gives the nervous system an indication: "This is the direction in which we are going to go." Also this traction gently engages and stretches the neck muscles lying above.

Add additional vectors by proceeding down the back with the first fingers of your hands almost touching. Avoid going over the spinous processes.

Along the way, feel for the natural curves of the spine and slow down just a little when you encounter any particularly tense places. Continue down the back, going all the way to the level of the third or fourth sacral segment. When you come to the lower lumbar region, lift up the little finger sides of your hands so that you don't bump over the iliac crests. Continue down the sacrum, emphasizing contact with the distal end of your first finger, first phalange. Do lighten up on pressure when you are gliding down the sacrum.

This fulcrum is one of the longest of all that you'll do. As you move down the back, pay attention to sustaining the stroke so that it forms one long, deeply relaxing, lengthening experience. Note the duration. You want to go slowly enough so that you can feel tension and so that the client can release it from inside out. Yet you don't want to go so slowly as to trigger the client's impatience.

This fulcrum should feel good—ideally really good. It doesn't take much pressure to do this well, it just takes skill and care.

Monitor for change to sense how well this fulcrum is working. Note changes in breathing. Particularly look for movements of the lower back as the client may positively respond by breathing in and out more fully.

Near the bottom of the sacrum, clearly disengage. End decisively on a note of length.

Repeating this fulcrum two or three times at the beginning of the session helps organize the client around his or her center and integrate the other freedoms you will be facilitating. During the session, when the client is prone, it is fine to repeat it anytime you feel it will be helpful.

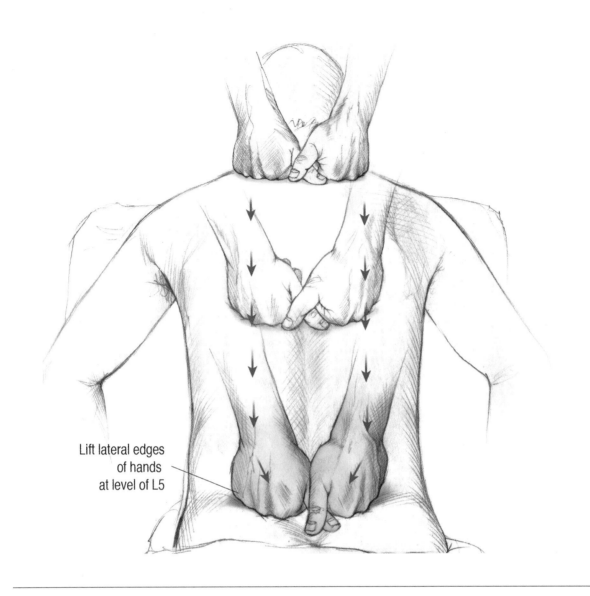

Lift lateral edges
of hands
at level of L5

Figure 1. Fists Down the Erectors

A NOTE ON HAND AND WRIST PLACEMENT

For most people's bodies, your most aligned position will be with the first finger sides of the fists almost touching and the little finger sides of your fists about 2" apart—so your hands are at about a 45° angle to each other. My extended thumbs usually overlap, making an "X." Your working surface is the proximal phalanges of your fingers, especially the fourth and fifth (shifting to the first as you approach the sacrum).

Interestingly, the lower back muscles are not very available from the back. They have many layers, each lying deeper than the last. Practically speaking, coming in from the side is the most direct way to access and address the lower back.

You will work into one side and then build the next fulcrum ("Ironing Up the Erectors") before going to the other side of the lower back.

Center yourself, remembering to stay as relaxed as you can during this fulcrum. In the beginning please do not press in hard or work with any unnecessary effort.

Excess pressure can be painful to your client and hurt your own wrists, fingers, or back. *Never substitute force for intelligence!*

Start while standing on the left side of the client. Place your right foot on the floor at the level of the client's thigh and your left foot more at the level of the pelvis. Take your right hand across the body to the right side of the lower back. Find the bony landmarks—the iliac crest and a few inches above it the 12th rib. Between them lies the lumbar musculature.

Position the fingers of your right hand at a 90° angle to your palm. Place the fingers, particularly the thumb-side of the first finger, snugly up against the lateral margin of the lumbar muscles. This hand will hold the right side of the lumbar muscles in place, creating stability, while your more active left hand will press into the left side of the lumbar muscles.

As you center yourself, assume a position standing alongside the client at the level of the thighs. The client will be face down, ideally with the head in the face cradle. With gently curved fingers, press in with your left hand just above the iliac crest and into the side of the erector spinae. You are pressing into the lateral margin of these muscles about 2" lateral to the spinous processes. Take out the looseness—pressing *onto* tension if it's present. Now with just a little more pressure, take up the slack, pressing *into* the tension a bit more deeply. It should feel good or at least neutral for your client. Your pressure is directed medially, toward the center.

You may find no tension or particular sensitivity. If so, great! Just clearly disengage. However, if you do feel some tension or the client reports you are on a relevant spot, then rest into the area, sinking in, creating a fulcrum. Then the client relaxes his or her own tension from inside out.

You may not notice any change, or you may feel a hard place melt and suddenly feel softer. Just hold the fulcrum and allow the client to release from inside out. Monitor for any overt signs of the client's letting go.

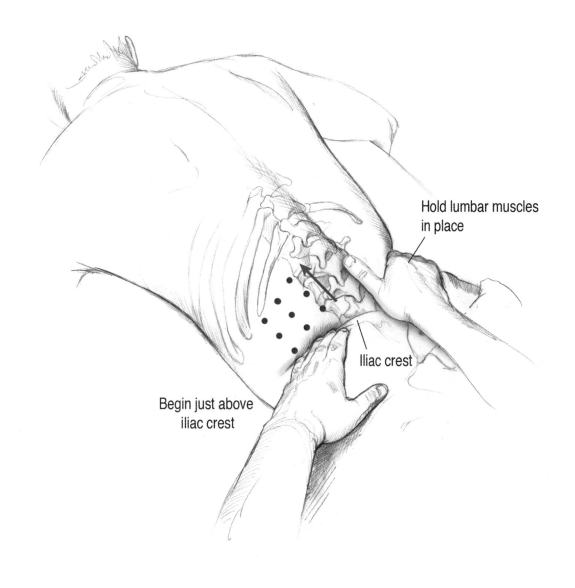

Figure 2. Nine Points

At any of the points here, usually three seconds is quite enough time. Better to err on the side of leaving the client wanting more, rather than feeling overworked, forced to change, or wanting less. Again if you find no tension, you will recognize that almost immediately and can clearly disengage without building the fulcrum.

Clearly disengage with the left hand. Allow the client a breath or two, then press into the next of the nine points. This will be halfway between the iliac crest and the 12th rib, again into the side of the erector group. Note these points are not anatomically landmarked. We have just chosen to address this fairly small but crucial area in detail, searching for and addressing low back tension just above the iliac crest, halfway between it and the 12th rib, and just underneath the 12th rib. Proceed as before. If you feel tension, rest in and build the fulcrum; if not, move on.

The third point is just below the 12th rib into the side of the erectors.

The fourth point is at the same level as the first, just above the iliac crest. It goes into a deeper muscle layer, the multifidus. To ensure your entry into the deeper layer, begin exploring with your left hand placed more laterally. Then, when you press in, you will be one layer deeper.

Again note these muscle layers are not anatomically distinct to palpation. The lower back muscles are like a 3" thick beefsteak. Use the illustration and these directions to give you a good sense of the layers you are addressing.

As above, in this fourth area, build a fulcrum if needed. Then again explore halfway between the iliac crest and the 12th rib; and finally just below the 12th rib. These are points 4-6.

The deepest layer of the lower back is the quadratus lumborum. To position yourself to access it properly, start still more laterally. Looking from the side, you are starting about a third of the way toward the front of the body.

Again press into the three points, building fulcrums as necessary, just over the iliac crest, halfway between it and the 12th rib, and then just below the 12th rib.

After you've done the next fulcrum, "Ironing Up the Erectors," you will repeat "Nine Points" on the right side.

Ironing Up the Erectors

I was once working with a client, making my way slowly up his mid-back with my forearm. He asked, "What are you working on?" I answered, "I'm just working up your ribcage." He replied, "I didn't know I had ribs in my back!"

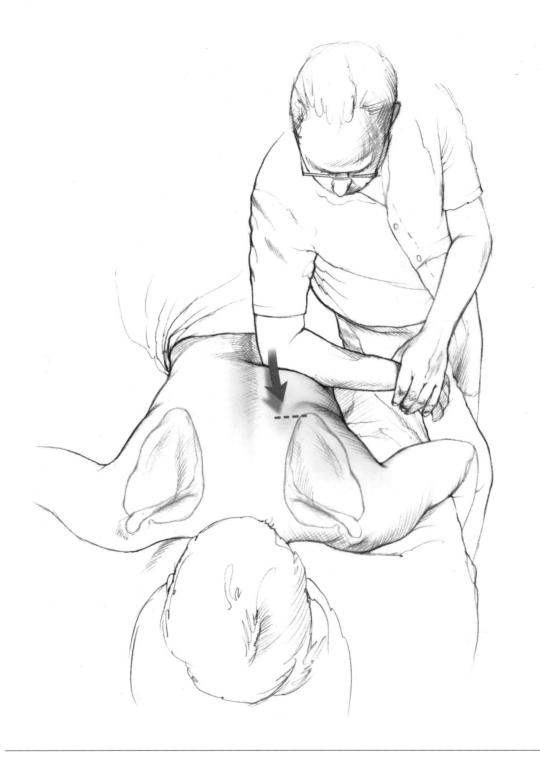

Figure 3. Ironing up the Erectors – 1

Many people suffer from a lack of knowledge of the workings and components of their own body. Philosopher and bodyworker Thomas Hanna called it "sensori-motor amnesia."

The broad surface of the back is composed mostly of ribs surrounded by soft tissue and housing the heart and lungs. To address the back we certainly need a fulcrum that will free the ribs and their associated tissues.

When I think of this fulcrum, I recall my Godmother, Millie Barry, showing me as a little boy how to iron. There was something both comforting and restorative about applying heat and pressure and care, watching as the wrinkled fabric acquired a lovely new smoothness.

At the end of a challenging day, it is common to feel one's back having born the stress of the day, perhaps leaving you feeling a bit bent out of shape.

In Deep Massage we work with clearer, stronger force fields than those currently in the body. Like ironing a shirt, we notice how clearer, stronger fields override disorganized structure and energy.

A touch that knows anatomy and engages the client with utmost clarity, through the steps of the fulcrum, reawakens the body part and the whole person to a clearer, stronger experience of themselves.

This fulcrum follows the nine points on the left side and is followed by nine points on the right and ironing up on the right.

Initially, your working tool here will be your forearm with elbow well bent, so that your hand is almost pointed at your own waist. Your forearm then will be generally perpendicular to the spine.

Starting on the left side of your client, center yourself; then stand facing towards the client's head, with your legs alongside the client's pelvis. The client will be lying prone. Place your forearm near the bottom of the ribcage around T11. Do not put pressure in but just take out the looseness, settling into the ribs and tissues here.

Now take up the slack, initiating a pulling of the tissues superiorly, prior to moving through the tissue.

Add additional vectors, ascending the back slowly. Proceed with care and curiosity. Sense the shape, tensions, and movements in the client's body.

Go slowly enough that you can feel the movement of breath—or lack thereof—between the ribs. In places where you sense more tension or less freedom, feel free to slow down, or to rest in and melt away the tension. Slowly, patiently, iron out the tension and help restore the natural, free excursion of ribs and soft tissues. Ultimately, you are helping to free the diaphragm, heart, and lungs as you create a more spacious and better organized surrounding environment.

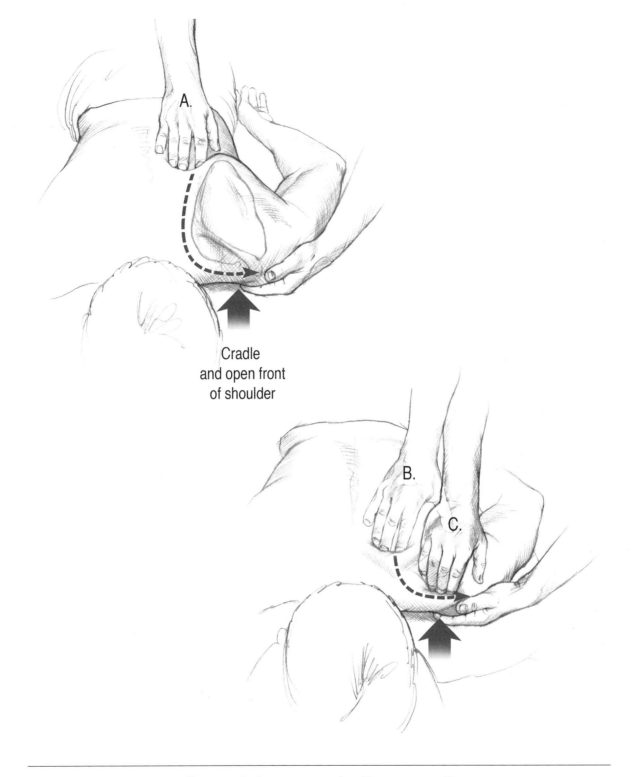

Cradle
and open front
of shoulder

Figure 4. Ironing up the Erectors – 2

When you reach the level of the scapula, at about T7 or T8, your forearm will run up against the bottom edge of the scapula. I have found continuing to work with the forearm or elbow between the scapulae to be problematic and have had at least one occasion where a student injured a client by working with the elbow near the base of the neck.

While working between the scapulae (Figure 4), gracefully change positions. Let your left hand disengage and cup the front of the shoulder. From this position, you can gently traction the front of the shoulder girdle open, pulling laterally, adding an even greater three-dimensionality to this fulcrum. Position your right hand, fingers gently spread, in the area between the scapula and the spine. Take out the looseness around T8. Take up the slack, initiating an upward pull. Then add additional vectors, slowly working up with your finger pads from T8 to T1.

It is irresistible to finish the second part of this fulcrum with the fingers of the right hand hooking into and pulling laterally through the trapezius and supraspinatus lying in the supraspinous fossa.

There is often so much tension between and above the scapulae that I repeat this fulcrum 2-3 times. Do whatever you sense you and your client feel is optimal.

And the hands go and go;
The sacred surfaces are smoothed.

— Pablo Neruda

Movement—the Second Dimension of Touch

Nature is the art of God.

— Dante Alighieri

On many levels, we are discovering that freedom is not something that can be "guaranteed" by a constitution. In recent centuries, calls to rise up and "loose our chains" have won us many precious external freedoms. Yet inner chains remain that can be equally binding.

I am profoundly aware in my own life, and have observed in all my clients and students, that the legacy of freedom promised by democracy means little without inner freedom. Enslavement to social roles, to family-transmitted neurotic patterns, to the limiting ideas and behaviors of profiteering and bureaucracy, to the unhealed wounds within

each of our biographies, to denying responsibility for one's own life—many of these limitations are as epidemic as ever. They cause the world and everyone in it deep pain.

In her book, **Rolfing,** Ida Rolf points out that challenges in our personal history may result in fascial restrictions that can cause our movements—both spiritually and physically—to be difficult in unnecessary ways. Massage practice beckons people to heal and free themselves. It reminds us that we have nothing to lose but our chains. The actual chains, ones we can touch, the points of maximum existential leverage, are to be found in our physical body.

In massage, as in dancing, we first touch, then move together. There is a certain resplendence, distinct and yet connected to these two ways of relating. When we clearly meet, an I-Thou relationship is established, one of mutual respect and trust. The therapist evokes the client's clear experience of contact, of illuminated one-dimensionality, by the laying on of a hand—what I refer to as the resting stroke.

This simple contact has an aura of the eternal and a majestic stillness. When we begin to move our hands, establishing a plane within the client's energy and structure, both client and therapist experience a heightened sense of two-dimensionality—the paths and the flows that constitute the self. With movement, we step out from the virtual into the actual world. As Buckminster Fuller said, "God is a verb." Or, as they say in the movies, "Action!"

With movement, we begin to co-create a story.

Anatomy and the Haptic Artist

To be moving intelligently within the body, we must know intimately the routes of being that nature has created within us. As a dancer knows how the body's parts coordinate with one another, as the painter knows pigments and the virtues of each brush, the therapist must have an intimate connection to the medium of his/her work—the living matter of humanity.

Of all the arts, ours is perhaps the only one in which the actual living substance of another's body, mind, and spirit makes up our explicit medium. Other arts address us through the more distal senses of sight and hearing. Massage at its highest level is purely a haptic art and science.

As haptic artists, we must be thoroughly familiar with our medium. If our movements reveal a lack of knowledge of the bodyscape, mistrust will automatically arise. With deep palpable knowledge, the client's energy meets that of the therapist. As we move together, we will be touching energy and structure simultaneously. In that clear moment, both therapist and client experience what Pehr Henrik Ling, founder of Swedish massage, made reference to when he said, "We ought to consider the organs of the body not as the lifeless forms of a mechanical mass, but as the living, active instruments of the soul."

If humans are indeed created in the image of God, then learning and feeling anatomy is literally to learn how to dwell consciously in the intricate, reflected presence of the divine.

Late in his life, I was honored to have discussions about haptic art with world-renowned architect Charles Moore. In his book, ***Body, Memory and Architecture,*** he wrote:

> *"The haptic sense is the sense of touch reconsidered to include the entire body rather than merely the instruments of touch, such as the hands. To sense haptically is to experience objects in the environment by actually touching them (by climbing a mountain rather than staring at it). Treated as a perceptual system, the haptic incorporates all those sensations (pressure, warmth, cold, pain, and kinesthetics) which previously divided up the sense of touch, and thus it includes all those aspects of sensual detection which involve physical contact both inside and outside the body. For example, if you accidentally swallow a marble you may haptically sense it as it moves through your body, thus experiencing part of the environment within your body. Similarly, you may sense body motion haptically by detecting movement of joints and muscle through your entire bodyscape.* **No other sense deals as directly with the three-dimensional world or similarly carries with it the possibility of altering the environment in the process of perceiving it; that is to say, no other sense engages in feeling and doing simultaneously.** *This action/reaction characteristic of haptic perception separates it from all other forms of sensing which, in comparison, come to seem rather abstract."*

Movement Creates Meaning

How fitting that the movements we make should be called "strokes," evoking the brush strokes of painters! With our movements we draw upon the deepest experiences of meaning that all art forms seek to embody. Our varied strokes compose an hour-long clearing and transformative experience. The sharp strokes of cross-fiber, long and broad effleurages, light strokes reminding us of wind, and the fiery strokes of myofascial release help create a sustained in-the-flesh art experience.

Composer Roger Sessions once said that over the performance of an entire symphony, one should be able to draw a single long phrase marking from the first note to the last. In the same fashion, a well-performed massage is experienced as a single gesture—one long, articulated, purifying movement.

A wonderful session resolves into a meaningfulness that, like a painting or a symphony, goes far deeper than words. Our in-the-flesh art form results in an actual change of being. Philosopher Karl Marx once said, "Philosophers have merely interpreted the world; however the task is to change it." With our strokes, we actually change the world. We move and are moved beyond words. This is the thrill and responsibility inherent in haptic art.

The breaking wave and the muscle as it contracts obey the same law.

— Dag Hammarskjold

Our Medium is Water

As we move our hands through an individual's being, varying the depths and pace from the rapid strokes of sports massage to a simple laying-on of our hands, another meaning of "stroke" surfaces. We are approximately 60% water; therefore the movements we make are basically in a liquid medium. Not only is the client mostly water, but the therapist is as well. Our movements amount to water touching water—we are in effect swimming when we touch. Everything that makes swimming graceful and efficient and compelling is also called for in our bodywork.

Coordinating breath and stroke, extending our body's full length, feeling and watching for the varied expressions of life as we move along—the rocky places, the tangled places, the living creatures of the deep (each muscle an undersea organ), the hot springs and the cooler pools, the stagnant waters, the warm jets of vitality, the sea's overall temperament—choppy, rolling, tidal, lapping.

Any time we visualize an adhesion or fibrosity as something solid, we are in trouble. We have locked our movements and proprioceptive expectations into a position of therapeutic standoff. If tissue is met as a solid needing to be broken down, it will defend itself by hardening. Rather, if we move with the awareness that everything we touch, as well as the empty space pervading it, is primarily dense liquid that we are swimming in together, the body tensions will yield.

Let the calm, calm blue waters
Wash through your soul
Passing right through you,
Like the smallest rose out of the hardest ground
Like a tiny hand reaching up for the sun.

— Los Lobos

The Path of Healing is Not Straight

Years ago, some anthropologists went to Africa to study a tribe that had experienced almost no contact with "civilization." The aim of the study was to determine the impact on the natives of seeing photographic images for the first time.

The anthropologists took photos of everything—the mountains, the tribal members, their dwelling places, utensils, animals. They showed these to the chief. He was shocked. Through the interpreter the anthropologists queried what he found most remarkable.

After an animated conversation, the interpreter announced that the chief was not amazed by any of things pictured in the photographs, which he had seen many times before. What most puzzled him was how the anthropologists had created such straight lines around the images. He was looking at the borders around the pictures! Living in nature, he had never seen straight lines before—because in nature there are no straight lines, only curves.

In doing massage, since we are working in nature and, particularly, mostly in water, when we move in straight lines we are moving unnaturally. Yet sometimes massage techniques are taught as linear. In massaging straight up the leg or pressing directly into a pressure point we will be addressing the structure in general, but certainly not in its specificity. Any actual living structure, carefully explored, reveals itself to be curved in shape and spontaneous in its actions. As a matter of fact, to the felt body, a straight line is experienced as automatic, as predictable, as an abstraction, since it exists only in the mind of the human! To the felt body, a curved line speaks in the spontaneous language of nature. In massage, where our straight lines begin to curve is where freedom begins.

The Anatomy of Liberation

Fascia, let us recall, is thixotrophic. A thixotrophic substance, like paint or clay, will become more fluid when it is moved about or heated — when movement within it is increased. Its fluidity depends on the forces acting within and around it. Insofar as our fasciae contain cells of varying natures — neurons, muscle cells, white blood cells, fibroblasts — they are alive.

These cells in turn are connected and coordinated through the circulating liquid and electrical intelligence of the endocrine and nervous systems. The fasciae are changeable, alive, and intelligent. What then are we feeling when we encounter tension? Far from dumb adhesions, we are feeling the articulate tensing of an intelligent organism.

When we first learn bodywork, we are usually taught that we relax muscles. Not so! Tensing is not done by muscles, neither is relaxation. Fundamentally, relaxation is a function of the nervous system. Muscles only relax if the nerves stop stimulating them. If we want a person to let go of tension, we must find a way to touch the nervous system.

How can we do this? The nervous system, particularly the autonomic, responds on the basis of memory and association. To help someone become free of tension, we must evoke appropriate associations in the limbic system, which will trigger a "relaxation response." This will differ from person to person on the basis of their constitution and history. It will also differ from moment to moment and place to place within the living waters of their body. In any case, it is vastly important to realize that, due to the organism-wide effect of the autonomic nervous system, when we evoke this response, it is never local, it is always global. We can't just relax a leg. This is why we don't need to touch every part of the body for every part to relax. We may massage locally, but our freeing effect is, delightfully, global.

How to most easily evoke this global liberation of the self? If we move into the body carefully, we notice a place where the body first resists. This is the nervous system's way of responding to the difference between someone's touch on the body vs. someone touching *in* the body.

The stretch reflex is a macro-immune response designed to harden the surface of the body and to repel any force that threatens to affect the body too hard or too fast. However, if we gently enter the client's space with a curving stroke, and by respectfully pausing and relaxing at the first sign of resistance, our input is felt as non-threatening. With only the slightest increase of pressure on our part, we are allowed in. At each level of entry, the nervous system reconsiders whether to interpret the movement as unsafe, in which case it will harden and resist, or as trustworthy, in which case a vital exchange is more and more deeply experienced.

I would recommend working through no more than one or two layers of this yielding at a time. Once structure and energy are both engaged, the healing process is underway and it is important for the therapist to let that follow its course. As Dr. Fritz Smith says, "Raise a flag and see who salutes."

People often ask about the effects of bodywork. "How long will this last?" Our work is lasting when our movements together result in learning. Learning is permanent, manipulation is temporary.

The writer Johann Wolfgang von Goethe said that art is long, life is short. Similarly, in this haptic art and science of massage, manipulation is short, but education is long. As we learn how to create this abiding sense of meaning and inner freedom through movement, massage will be appreciated for its unique evolutionary leverage point. Once we can truly appreciate liberation through movement, we all can embody the freedom critical to our continuance and progress as individuals and as a species.

> *Your very flesh shall be a great poem,*
> *And have the richest fluency,*
> *Not only in its words,*
> *But in the silent lines of its lips and face,*
> *And between the lashes of your eyes,*
> *And in every motion and joint of your body.*
>
> *— Walt Whitman*

Posterior Pelvis and Back of Legs— Anatomy, Energy, and Fulcrums

The Pelvis

The pelvis and legs connect with the ground, with the whole Earth. With the pelvis, legs, and feet, we make our way through life, literally and figuratively choosing the paths along which we will walk.

The pelvis itself enfolds a wonderland of structure and energy: from the miraculously irregular structure of the bones— each side of the pelvis looks like two slightly twisted elephant ears—to the varied functions of elimination, procreation, birth, and balance. The pelvis is the connector, acting as the cornerstone of the upper and lower body. It houses our center, called the *dan tien* in Chinese, and *hara* in Japanese.

Despite its importance, or perhaps because of it, people have the most mixed of feelings regarding the pelvis. Shame and fear are common. Many individuals periodically dream of being naked or insufficiently clothed in public, where others will observe them unclothed.

Lovemaking and its anticipation— among life's most ecstatic pleasures—is also centered in the pelvis. The rhythmic swaying of the pelvis in dance or eros is infinitely enjoyable. Consider as well that its invaluable role in genesis has given the pelvic region a place of high regard both in art and culture. Our knowledge and our bodywork can help it retain the value and honor it deserves in our lives.

The Legs

When I think of the legs, I can hear Bob Marley's voice singing, *"Get up! Stand up! Stand up for your rights."* The legs play a fundamental role in our lives, although they rarely call attention to themselves. Yet it is often in the legs that we clearly see the most fundamental of energy imbalances.

In modern society, the upper half of the body gets vastly more attention and energy than the lower half. We emphasize education of the mind to the extent that some people barely are aware of having legs—until they develop a problem. This upward focus of attention to the mind or to our faces is often accompanied by a heightened concern with the appearance of our upper body and face. We tend to identify ourselves with our face most of all.

However, the manner in which we use our legs can be as revealing of who we are as the words we say or our facial expressions.

Melting into the Gluteus Maximus

With the client face down on the table, place a bolster under the client's ankles.

Breathe in and out fully. Center yourself. Stand alongside the left side of the pelvis, your feet shoulder-width apart, and face the client's knees. Bend your left elbow to nearly 90°, letting your right hand rest gently on the back of your left wrist. You will be working into the center of the large muscle overlying the back of the pelvis, the gluteus maximus.

Using the proximal surface of the forearm beneath the elbow (spanning 3-4 inches below your elbow), make your initial contact into the center of the muscle. With interface established, press gently toward the table surface and take out the looseness. Take up the slack with just a bit more pressure in the same direction.

It may feel like you are gracefully floating down through water. Continue breathing fully, relaxing your belly, pelvis, and legs as much as possible. Now fine-tune your pressure, adding a slightly downward/inferior or outward/lateral vector, and hold it... hold it... hold it... giving the client a chance to deeply let go of the tension often held in this place.

When you sense "this is long enough," or see a working sign, clearly disengage and give the client a moment to integrate the experience.

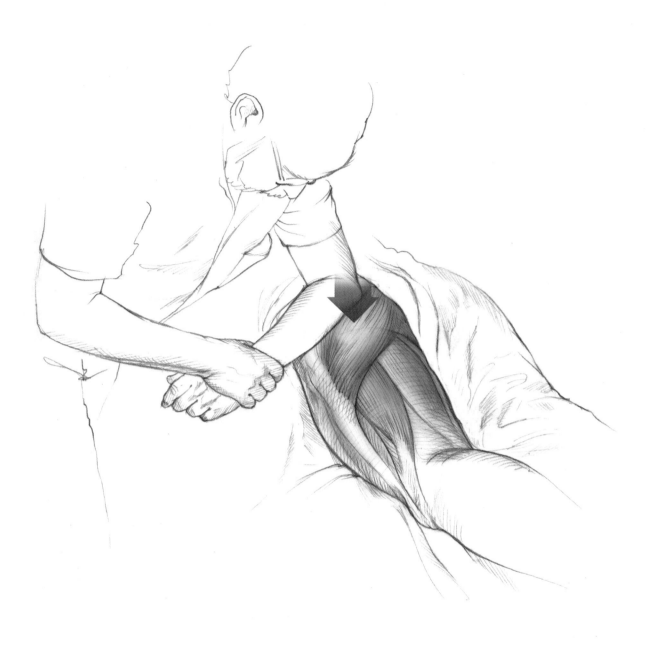

Figure 5. Melting into Gluteus Maximus

Lengthening the Gluteus Maximus

Stand along your client's side to begin working with the length of the gluteus maximus. For this stroke you will make three passes. Your primary working surface for the left leg will be the loose fist of your left hand, with an option for using your right hand on the third pass.

The first stroke starts on the back of the pelvis near the sacrum. It follows the curve of the gluteus maximus (usually shaped much like a large inverted teardrop), and ends on the side of the lower thigh about ¾ of the way down.

The second stroke starts about 2 inches more laterally and ends in the same place as the first.

The third stroke starts another 2 inches more laterally, almost on the side of the pelvis and thigh, and has the same ending place as the other two. In the case of this third stroke you have the option to switch hands, placing your left on the back of the sacrum to gently traction down the whole spine, while lengthening the pelvis and leg with the loose fist of the right hand facing up.

Often people have a sense of the back of their pelvis as being a broad fleshy area unconnected to their movement. In fact, the gluteal muscles are the primary muscles enabling our forward momentum. Just like a horse, we extend our hips forcefully with these muscles. The gluteals are among the longest muscles in the body, running from the very top of the pelvis to just above the knee.

When they contract, they exert great leverage on the thigh and therefore are, energetically as well as physically, a primary source of propulsion in our lives. Amplifying the client's sense of these muscles as beautiful, long, strong, and powerful is much of what we hope to accomplish here.

Center yourself, breathing and relaxing into your legs and your whole body. Stand alongside the left leg, feet shoulder-width apart, at a slight angle to the body, facing toward the feet.

Place your left loose fist just next to the sacrum and just below the top of the pelvis. Press in, anteriorly, taking out the looseness. Take up the slack, changing the angle of your fist to aim your traction downward (foot-ward).

Begin following the muscle down in two vectors, foot-ward and toward the side. Proceed mindfully down, ending on the outside of the thigh about three-quarters of the way down. During this stroke your right hand can rest either lower down the leg or on the table surface, whichever feels better. Then clearly disengage.

Now place your left loose fist just below the top of the pelvis about one-and-a-half to two inches lateral to your first starting point. Follow the steps of the fulcrum as in the previous pass.

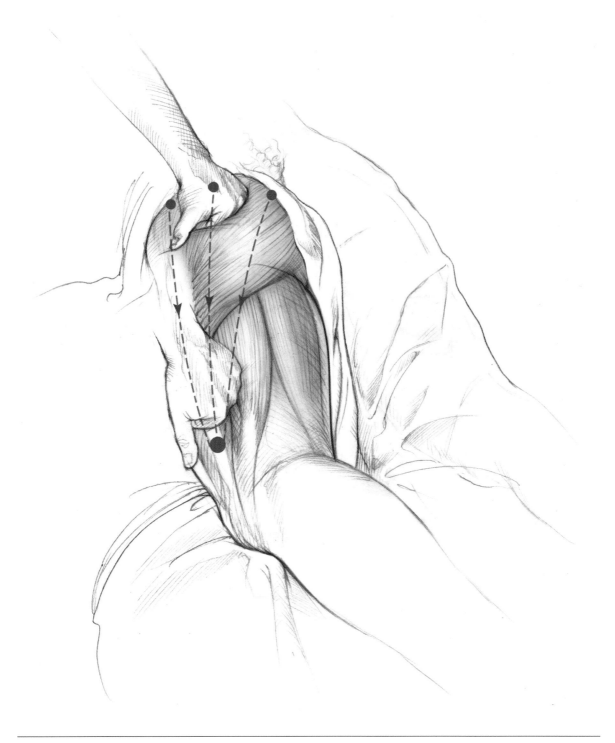

Figure 6. Lengthening Gluteus Maximus

Your ending place is again the same one as in the first stroke, the outer surface of the thigh about three-quarters of the way down.

You can choose to do the third pass two different ways. One is with the left fist as the primary working tool, starting just 1.5 inches more lateral than the second pass. Follow the pathway of the other two strokes.

An option (not shown in Figure 6) is to place the palm of your left hand over the back surface of the sacrum. Have your left palm aligned with the spine, not at an angle. Simultaneously place your _right_ loose fist palm up below the top of the pelvis about 1.5-2 inches lateral to the last starting point.

Take out the looseness using both hands, the left gently stretching the lower back, the right pressing into the gluteal muscles. Then generally follow the steps as outlined above for the first two fulcrums for lengthening the gluteus maximus.

In either case, with the third pass over the hip, you will want to ease up slightly as you go over the greater trochanter—the bony upper surface of the thigh. As you continue the stroke with the right fist, you may want to gently traction the sacrum/lower back just a little more. This not only amplifies the feeling of elongating the pelvis and leg, but, by engaging the whole spine, deepens the sense of total body-lengthening and letting go.

Hamstrings

You will first be working with the loose fist of your left hand. To get a little extra looseness into this tendinous area you will, with your right hand supporting the client's ankle, work with the knee bent to about 90°. This fulcrum proceeds from the sitz bones to the lower leg just below the back of the knee. You will make three strokes, each starting at the common origin, the ischial tuberosity, and proceeding down the outer, middle, and inner surfaces of the back of the thigh.

Before beginning the stroke, center yourself; relax your body and breathe. Place your right palm under the client's ankle and lift the leg gently to 90°. Take the loose fist of your left hand, thumb side facing down toward the feet, and make a good contact with the bottom of the "sitz" bone (the ischial tuberosity of the pelvis). Take out the looseness. Take up the slack, tractioning the tissue here slightly toward the feet. Now begin moving in two vectors, down and slightly outward (through the biceps femoris).

Continue slowly and confidently down the thigh, ending finally on the back of the fibula just below the knee. When you go behind the knee, to finish the stroke on the back of the fibula, you naturally change the angle of your fist to be thumb-side facing upward. Then clearly disengage.

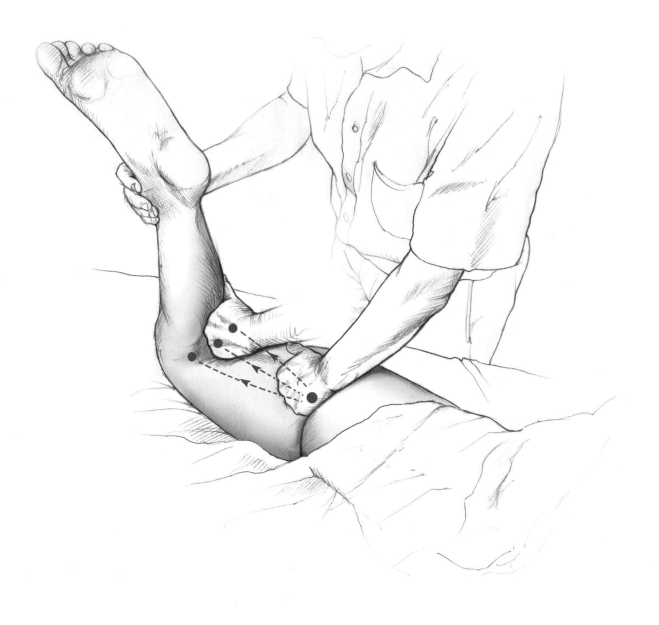

Figure 7. Hamstrings

Begin again at the sitz bones. Follow the steps outlined above, but this time take a path basically straight down the back of the thigh. I find this fulcrum works even better if I position the loose fist so that I'm working with the ridge of "knuckles" between the proximal and intermediate phalanges.

As you get near the knee, be sure to ease up considerably with your pressure, as there are important vessels and nerves near the surface here. Again with slight pressure, end just below the knee. Clearly disengage.

Begin at the sitz bones again and follow the steps as outlined above, proceeding along the medial surface of the back of the thigh. Continue down to the back of the tibia, ending just below the knee at the attachment of the semimembranosus. Clearly disengage.

Gently lower the leg back to the table surface and give the client a few moments to assimilate the experience.

Gastrocnemius and Soleus

Assuming you will work on the back of the left leg first, stand alongside the client's knee. Place a bolster under the client's ankles. Position your feet shoulder-width apart, facing the foot. Center yourself.

For this fulcrum, you can use the distal end of your right arm, with the right ulna being your main working surface and your left palm pushing against the radial side of the arm. Sometimes that slightly concave surface of the distal ulna works better in terms of meeting the client's shape here, as well as facilitating easier body mechanics. This fulcrum will proceed from just below the knee to the sole of the foot.

Alternatively, you can bend your left arm to about 90° so that the elbow is pointing away from you. Your left hand is close to your solar plexus and your right hand rests gently on the back of your left hand.

You will be working with the bony surface of your left forearm a few inches below the elbow.

Center yourself, breathing and letting your weight relax into your legs. Using the proximal surface of your forearm, press into the client's lower leg just below the knee and take out the looseness. Take up the slack, aiming foot-ward. Begin to move down following the curving surface of the calf, maintaining your pressure while carefully monitoring the client's comfort as you proceed.

Continue this lengthening at a leisurely pace until you reach the Achilles tendon. Slow down even more, giving the tendon time to lengthen and soften as you go. Proceed gently along the tendon onto the back surface of the heel bone.

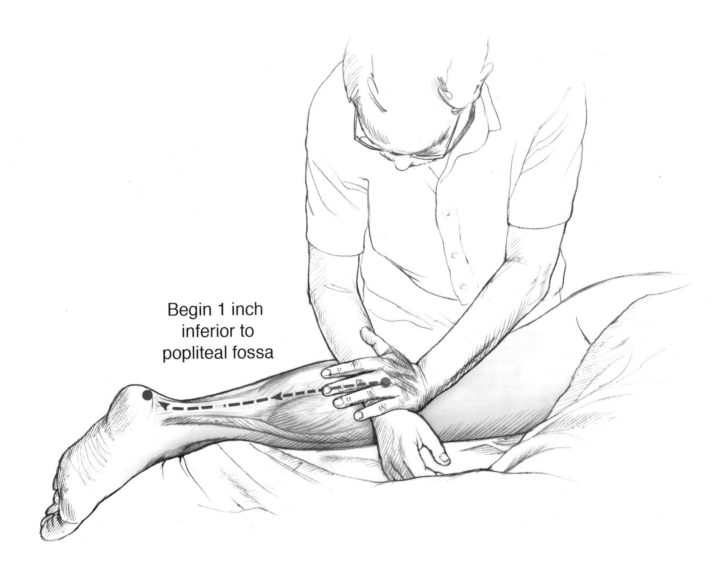

Begin 1 inch
inferior to
popliteal fossa

Figure **8.** Gastrocnemius and Soleus

Notice, through your leverage on the heel bone, how you can gently traction the entire body by pressing inferiorly on the posterior surface of the calcaneus. Slow down even more to allow for the whole body to lengthen as you proceed across the surface of the posterior calcaneus. Then rest when you get to its end. Clearly disengage. Give the client a moment to themselves in which to assimilate this new experience.

Breath—The Third Dimension of Touch

As noted, in the last twenty years more progress has been made in the realm of touch than at any other time in history. This is a phenomenal cultural and evolutionary event. The proliferation of modalities arising from new theories and practices is both inspiring and bewildering, much as the sudden appearance of a thousand butterflies.

The predominant development in the therapeutic landscape over the last ten years has been linked to our anatomical coming of age. Sports massage, deep tissue massage, myofascial release, trigger point work—these and other approaches owe their popularity to the practitioner's skill and frequent brilliance in applying advanced anatomical knowledge. Many therapists are now competent, if not expert, in their ability to understand and respond to the needs of human structure.

The strength of these structural approaches has allowed us to put our work on a solid scientific footing and thus help our clients more effectively. The limitation is that there is more to people than just their structure. They are also energetic, feeling, thinking, and spirited beings. A strictly structural approach is therefore not effective in relieving tensions that may arise from feelings, thoughts, and restricted energy flows. Any time we imagine we are merely working on muscular tissue, we have dehumanized the person and put our efficacy as practitioners into jeopardy.

I believe we are now seeing and participating in a new and appropriate phase of our growth, one that will be perhaps even more exciting and fruitful than our achievements in anatomical understanding. This new phase is the conscious development of knowledge and skill with regard to the energetic aspect of bodywork. In our present world, needs beyond the structural are crying out to be competently addressed.

Until recently our culture has defined progress mostly in terms of structure, technique, and training—the software of intellectual understanding, the hardware of machines and manufactured products. This chronic over-emphasis on technology has exacerbated our ever more desperate need is to address the unanswered question: how shall we live? How can we optimize a healthy relation to ourselves and the natural environment of which we are a part?

Our answer is: through being in touch.

Touch therapy heightens physical experience, helps us attain a new emotional balance, vitalizes the spirit, and inspires new thoughts on the appropriate relation of nature, mind, emotion, body, and spirit.

Touch is unconsciously identified as a source of solutions to fundamental issues humanity must now address if we are to survive and hopefully thrive.

Thus the incredible momentum propelling the rise of sophisticated touch therapy is explicable because it is advancing our evolution as whole beings, not just technological automatons. If this therapeutic opportunity were restricted to massage as a structural, orthopedic modality it would be a tragedy of historic proportions.

Let us enthusiastically accept our good fortune—the opportunity to evolve new ways of being in touch with ourselves and in touch with the world.

An enlightened experience of being-in-touch recognizes the ways we are connected subjectively and objectively. Even though touch takes place in space, it has many more dimensions than those comprised by the three spatial axes. Refined qualities of touch also convey new worlds of sensation, feeling, intuition, and insight. Each dimension of touch has a structural and energetic aspect.

When we initially touch the body, establishing a one-dimensional point of contact, where and how we lay our hands can convey radically new ways to meet each other with compassion, curiosity, and courage. Where and how we then move our hands, establishing two-dimensional planes of movement, can illuminate how we are structured and enhance energy flows along the pathways of our being.

The Source of Our Work Is Not Our Hands

The third dimension of bodywork arises from the miracle of breath. The life-defining expansion and contraction of breath fuels and refreshes every cell in the body. Each time we heighten our capacity to breathe—through our therapeutic impact on the nervous and endocrine systems, the muscles and fascia that define the excursion of our lungs, and all other bodily tissues—we facilitate more oxygen delivery, and enhance and enliven every cell in our body.

This is energy work! We don't need to get esoteric to understand energy work. Let us expand our understanding of energy work beyond the arcane obscurity of some of its devotees. Every enlivening breath helps open us up to greater life, greater vitality. Each exhale lets go of unneeded metabolic and energetic waste products — emotional tensions, old patterns of thought and feeling, and habitual behaviors. The carbon dioxide we exhale is made available to the plant kingdom.

Trees have a structural and energetic role as the lungs of the earth. We human animals, having the tree-like structures of our bronchioles, participate in the grandeur of this planetary breath exchange.

It is easy to overlook the amplitude of breath as an energy source. We take an average of 20,000 breaths each day. Compare this frequency to our consumption of food and drink. Perhaps every book on nutrition should begin with a chapter on breath!

We are used to thinking that we do bodywork with our hands. To teach about breath as a part of good "body mechanics" misses the deeper point. While it is true our hands are the structures we most commonly use to contact the body, they are not our essential energy source. It is from our breath that energy flows into our hands.

Hands are the structural tools for our work. Breath is our fundamental energetic tool. Breath is the "origin"; hands are the "contact."

Breath as Autonomic Modulator

Holistic bodywork leaves out nothing. Since people aren't actually divided into parts, we cannot but work with the whole. We work with body, emotions, mind, and spirit. Breath is one of the primary access points to spirit. Unlike the heartbeat, for example, which is fundamental but not under the control of the conscious mind, with breath we are given the unique opportunity of conscious control of one of the deepest actions within ourselves. Through conscious breathing we can modulate the autonomic nervous system. We can fine-tune our spirit through breath.

Breath, while personal, is not experienced in the realm of ego. It is deep inside us but not of us. As we breathe, we take in from the outside and give out to the outside. Quite simply and profoundly, the experience of breath amounts to a life-giving movement of air through us. It is for this reason that many meditation techniques instruct us to focus on the breath. To the extent that we place our awareness on breath, we move beyond ego. Living beyond narrow self-centeredness is a central theme within all spiritual disciplines.

Breath then is an avenue to autonomic self-modulation and a direct-access way to the spiritual. As therapists wanting to invest our spirit fully in our work, we bring ourselves into an honored, conscious awareness of breath before we begin each session. This intimacy, this alignment with our own spirit, continues throughout the session as we breathe easily and fully.

The Experience of Three-Dimensionality

Most people experience themselves as having only two dimensions, a front and a back, both with height and width. They know they have a front because they see it in the mirror. They know they have a back because it hurts sometimes. Another structure that has a front and a back is a piece of paper. In their self-image such individuals experience themselves as having no more depth than a piece of paper.

The self-imaging of their body structure as two-dimensional is itself a source of disease. Firstly, the image is out of sync with three-dimensional physical reality. Secondly, on an energetic level, if we do not feel depth within ourselves, we experience a diminished capacity for emotion, because emotion requires a sense of spaciousness, or internal room to move. In an experientially two-dimensional world, the organs themselves lack enough room to function optimally.

The key to the therapist and client experiencing their dimensional depths is breath. Breath, with its unceasing rhythm of in and out, is the most dramatic experience we have of three-dimensionality. When we slow down, we sense the three-dimensional tidal movement of inhaling, becoming larger, feeling our borders widen, broaden, and deepen. On exhaling we sense the out-rushing air and our boundaries easing in toward center. The three-dimensional waving and pulsating that breath continually presents to us, accompanied by the pulsing of our beating heart, is a primary way we know we are alive.

As therapists it is imperative that we fully inhabit our three-dimensionality and pulsation through a conscious and enthusiastic relationship with breathing. Firstly we energize ourselves through the effects of heightened cellular respiration. Secondly we let go of held tension in our bodies, so as to move more effectively and impart a tone of ease to the session. Thirdly we set a therapeutic example for the client. Your breath as a therapist gives assent and blessing to the breathing aliveness of your client. Watch the client virtually inhale your permission to inhabit their living three-dimensionality, communicated purely by your breathing.

Hold your breath and touch yourself. Notice what is lacking. In various ways, a touch without sufficient breath feels un-alive: unmoving, not waving, not caring. There is a sense of waiting. Without breath we really haven't begun. Just as in the birth process, we joyfully anticipate the infant's first breath. When it starts, we rejoice as the waves of new life begin! We feel care, presence, the promise and spontaneity of relationship.

We don't and can't touch with just a part of ourselves because we are not divided. We touch with all of us. A fundamental aspect of touching is the breathing—the re-inspiration and the "ex-spiration" of our beings that takes place within a conscious breathing atmosphere. Thus we are able to see how fundamentally doing therapy is breath touching breath.

I add my breath to your breath that our days may be long on the Earth, that the days of our people may be long, that we shall be as one person, that we may finish our road together.

— Laguna Pueblo people

Palpation with Air

Too often we imagine that the client's restrictions are things we have to remove through force. We can fall into an earth-mover/bodyworker approach, plowing the fields of flesh in an attempt to re-route the fascia. Structural work can tend naturally to emphasize this way of working. But imagining the body as a fascial substance that we need to remodel gives rise to unnecessary conflict within and between the therapist and the client.

Previously we have noted that in substance we are mostly water, and that this water itself is mostly empty space. The ratio of empty space to matter in an atom is the same as the ratio of empty space to stars in the universe. The most tangible experience we have of this open space is through breath. When we have the experience that air is in a fundamental sense what we are, we become vastly more conscious of the open space inside us which constitutes our reality more deeply than the blip on the mind screen that is our conscious ego.

As a therapist you can communicate this essential experience and insight to your client by breathing freely, then touching with the imagery that you are both breath—breath touching breath. When we breathe freely, we palpate with the imagery of touching air, and thus heighten the client's perception of their own pulsating aliveness. We are working in a manner that is both structurally more accurate and energetically more connected.

Your hands energetically and structurally modify the fundamental energy of breath, in much the same manner as your mouth, teeth, and tongue shape the air column of breath into speech and song. In Hindu philosophy, sacred shapings of the hands are known as *mudras*. We can view each beautiful shape the hand makes of the breath in energetic touch as a healing *mudra*.

When we touch with the air element, our touch is all-perfusing, in the sense of fresh air flowing into a region. Consciously breathing, we bring air into our touch so as to penetrate without effort. We use our hands to shape and direct this energy as beautifully and powerfully as a singer shapes each moment of a song, as the poet savors the sound and profound meaning of each word. With this spiritual and aesthetic attention the client will experience change naturally and almost effortlessly.

This way of working evokes Gandhi's manner of encouraging political change: *Satyagraha*, meaning "soul force" or "insistence on truth," is a concept pivotal to his advocacy of non-violence. What a privilege it is to approach the body with soul force! Often the tensions we find are those created by the structural and energetic violence committed against us and by us. The soul force of breath shows us a way to end the violence against our beings, the traces of energetic and physical injuries, that we all hope to heal with this thrilling work of ours.

Window to the Spirit

We have noted that the eyes have long been considered the windows to the soul. The intimacy sensed when looking into another's eyes stems from soul-to-soul contact. The joy of gazing eye-to-eye is a sign of love. Even more intimate is the contact of breath-to-breath. At a personal level, this is usually reserved for friends and loved ones. A prolonged hug, curling up with a partner, noticing the sleeping breath of your pet or your child—these are experiences of profound connection.

At a professional level, the therapist feels with their hands and sees with their eyes the breathing of the client. From moment to moment it changes—slowing into sleep, breaking rhythm with a sigh like a cresting wave, breathlessly talking with excited insight, shaking when the client experiences the gently insistent surfacing of emotion. Clearly the breath is a window to the spirit.

As therapists, once we are aware of this, our gaze and our touching are transformed. Just as in the Biblical story of Creation, as we work, we can observe if "it is good." The client's breathing indicates how the spirit is being affected. Through it we can track the paths of being that the client explores in the course of the session. When we touch breath-to-breath, sensing the moment-to-moment shifts of being, both therapist and client are alive fully in the presence of spirit. It is—in the therapeutic sense—an act of love as palpable and real as a song in the open air.

As we feel the waves of being, the living swells and tides of breath controlled both consciously and unconsciously, we fully experience that we are alive. Breath reminds us that being alive is a continuous miracle.

The rhythms of living breath inform the rhythms of our hands and our body movements. They synchronize feelings, thoughts, and being, giving rise to a profound body-work/bodymind experience. When we participate in this rhythm together we experience a moment together, the infinite life that we share.

"Between the conscious and unconscious the mind has put up a swing," wrote the Indian poet, Kabîr. As we swing with our focus through the vast dimensions of being—the structures, consciousness, feelings, energy flows, spirit—we know we are not alone. We are all on a great swing. WE ARE ALL ONE WAVING WORLD.

The waving that carries on through us reminds us that we can neither divide ourselves into parts—feelings here, body there—nor can we truly divide the outer world into parts—air here, fire there. Everything is connected and swinging. From a rigorous physics view of energy, the universe is one incredibly complex waveform.

The Legs: Front and Sides—
Anatomy, Energy, and Fulcrums

Structure and Energy

The legs support the pelvis, torso, shoulder girdle, arms, head, and neck. They balance and ground us on the earth and give us the ability to stand, walk, and run. Legs provide vitality and nourishment for the whole self in the sense that we feel dramatically energized by a vigorous walk. Healthy legs feel alive, sensual, strong, and handsome or beautiful in an animalistic way.

The legs and feet also amplify or express our capacity for excitement. Note how children run not for exercise but in response to the irrepressible excitement of life.

Think of the legs as the southern hemisphere, a refreshing counterpoint to the usual realm of ceaseless ruminations in the north, the head. Our economy and education incline us to overvalue the brain and

conscious thought and to undervalue feelings, spirit, and the body. Massaging the legs—because they are literally the furthest from the head—is one of the most powerful ways to address this imbalance and to bring a person's awareness out from its reclusive, imbalanced attic residence and back into the whole body and self.

In yogic thought, the energetic character of the feet, legs, and base of the pelvis relates to the first *chakra*—one of the body's seven centers of spiritual power. This has been traditionally associated with survival as well as grounding. Notice how your pelvic floor may unconsciously tighten with reflexive fear when you peer out over the edge of a precipice.

Unreleased anxieties fostered by early life experiences, everyday stresses, the pace of modern life, and even the scare tactics of much of our news media can lead to chronic tension throughout the body. Often a fight-or-flight response is expressed through the legs, or when emotion is repressed, through their tension.

Relaxing the legs greatly reduces the overall anxiety level of the person. Letting go in the legs allows us to relax more into our animal nature and our connection to the earth. We relax into our deeper self, into the structural and energetic foundation of our being.

This area of the body also may suffer from what Thomas Hanna referred to as sensori-motor amnesia. People will use their legs like vehicles to get them from one place to another while remaining otherwise unconscious of them. Allowing oneself to feel the legs as a deeply personal, alive place is a revelation for most people.

All the above applies to the therapist as well. Especially relevant for the therapist's use of the legs is an application of Ida Rolf's wonderful insight, "Gravity is the therapist." In Deep Massage it is of fundamental importance to avoid deriving pressure through effort from the hands, arms, or shoulder girdle. It is always preferable, whenever possible, to derive pressure by using gravity. This means placing the hands on the client's body, relaxing your legs, leaning in or sinking in a little earthward so that pressure comes from gravity and the relaxation of your legs and not from the tensing of your upper body muscles. As I often say to students, "You have a choice. You can work by constantly recruiting your muscular system or you can work effortlessly with the freely available gravitational force of an entire planet. Which do you choose?"

Structurally, Deep Massage will have a dramatic impact on compression of the hip, hyperextension of the knees, overall joint compression throughout the leg, and pronation and supination of the ankle. It will help prevent hamstring pulls, calf cramps, shin splints, and any excess muscle tension or adhesion in this region. Should problems develop, working with the foundation of our structure and energy is part of any good session plan. It is also important that well-timed Deep Massage be included in the healing process of trauma to the legs or feet, as long as it is not contraindicated. The restoration of length to the muscles and fascia and the relaxation of the nervous system are critical for full recovery.

Rectus Femoris/Vastus Intermedius

For this main stroke on the leg, stand alongside the client's pelvis facing the feet. If you will be working on the client's right leg, let your right leg be forward of your left, about shoulder-width apart, with most of your weight on the right.

Bend your left arm to about 90° so that the elbow is pointing away from you. Your left hand is close to your solar plexus and your right hand can rest gently on the back of your left hand.

Center yourself. Breathe. Remember that your energy comes primarily from your breath—not your arm! Breathe freely and continuously throughout this stroke. The structural, working surface you will use is your forearm two to three inches below (distal to) your elbow. Place this part of your forearm in front of the client's hip joint. The coming into interface should not be abrupt, yet not so slow as to convey hesitation.

Relax your legs, bending your knees just a little, and sink gently into the front of the hip. Take out the looseness in the front of the hip joint by this gentle sinking in toward the table surface.

Next, without moving your arm, direct your pressure toward the feet as well, by leaning just a little more into your right leg. In this way you take up the slack in the front of the hip. The muscles you are now primarily contacting are the rectus femoris and, deep to it, the vastus intermedius.

Clearly maintaining your pressure and direction, begin slowly to move down the curving surface of the front of the thigh. The two vectors present in your movement are the pressing into the body and the downward stroking. The tempo here should be balanced, just as the coming to interface—not too fast, not too slow—what is sometimes called "the Goldilocks principle."

Sustain your general pressure, depth, and direction along the midline of the front of the thigh. As you get closer to the knee-cap, you may place your right hand gently on the knee, so the client is assured that you will not "run over" their kneecap. Continue the stroke until you reach the area just above (superior to) the kneecap. Fine tune as you go, attuning your awareness to what you feel and how the client is reacting. You may need to ease up slightly in a sore place or slow down as you encounter a little more tension.

When you reach the area an inch above the knee, pause, holding the traction and melting in. Then clearly disengage and give the client a moment to experience their thigh in a new way. This stroke can feel as if the tension has been squeezed out of the thigh like toothpaste out of a tube.

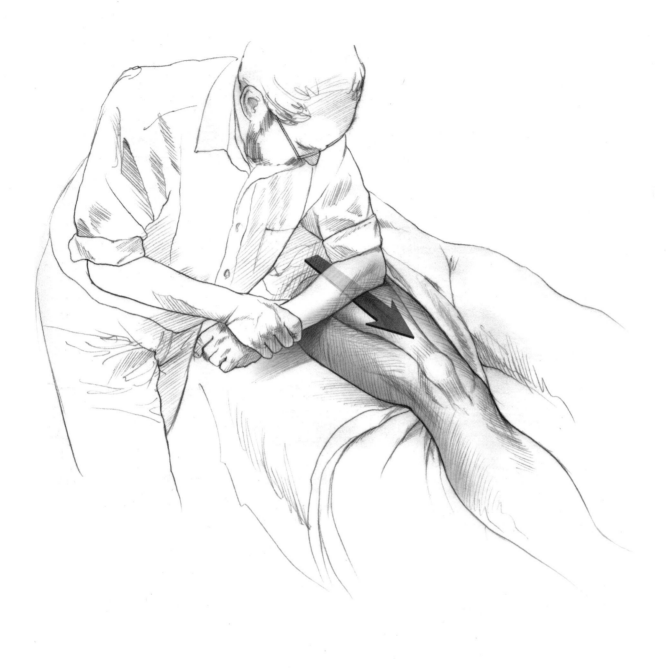

Figure 9. Rectus Femoris/Vastus Intermedius

Quadriceps Tendon/Patellar Ligament

This next simple stroke feels surprisingly good and can have profound energetic effects. Center yourself as you begin. If you are breathing somewhat shallowly, re-access your breath so your touch is fully oxygenated.

Standing alongside the client's lower leg, place the pads of your thumbs just above the kneecap at the midline of the thigh. Bring your awareness to this place as well so that you are now at interface. Soften your knees and use gravity for sufficient pressure to take out the looseness in the soft tissue above the kneecap. Now take up the slack in the soft tissue, stretching laterally and medially, preparing the thumbs to move down the outer and inner thigh.

Move your thumbs through the soft tissue laterally and medially so that you basically follow a line above the kneecap. Continue about a third of the way around the thigh so that you are then to the sides of the thigh just above the level of the kneecap. Pay close attention to your pressure, pace, and direction, and to the client's reaction. Note working signs if present. Clearly disengage. Pause for a brief moment. Now repeat.

Place your thumbs just beneath the kneecap—between the patella and the tibial tuberosity. Follow the same steps as above, stroking deeply from the midline in either direction. Clearly disengage, pause, and repeat.

Unless people have knee problems, they can be unaware of how much tension is often present around the knee. This stroke is a fantastic and simple way to erase that tension, awaken awareness of this important place, and restore a feeling of health and deep ease to an important, often neglected area of the body.

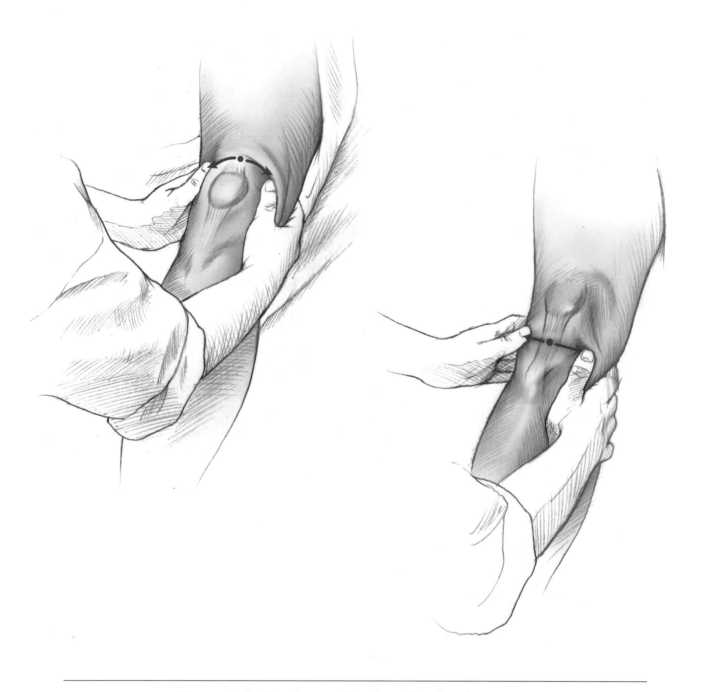

Figure **10.** Quadriceps Tendon/Patellar Ligament

The Deep Massage Book

Tensor Fascia Lata, Gluteus Medius, and Gluteus Minimus

The muscles on the side of the pelvis keep our hips level each time we lift a leg. When you lift your right leg to take a step forward, the muscles on the left side of pelvis automatically tense up, thus keeping the pelvis horizontal. They work so well that we are ordinarily unaware of the role they play in every single step we take.

This next fulcrum gives a neglected and hard-working part of us some long-overdue attention and care.

Start by sitting down on a chair or stool or kneeling, facing the side of the client's pelvis. Center yourself and remember to get most of your pressure by leaning into the person and leveraging gravity, not by pushing with your shoulder girdle.

You will be working into seven areas in the side of the pelvis while rotating the thigh inward. What you are doing in this stroke is creating a local softening in the side of the pelvis, accompanied by a freeing and opening of the hip joint itself.

Relax yourself and engage your breathing for the duration of this fulcrum. Place your left thumb into the soft tissue in the area just behind the top and front of the pelvic bone (in toward the surface of the ilium just behind the anterior superior iliac spine). This is the origin of the tensor fascia lata. Place the fingers of that hand gently on the lateral lower abdomen. Now place your right hand two-thirds of the way down the side of the thigh so that your right forearm rests on or near the table surface and the heel of the hand rests on the side of the thigh near the table surface, posterior to the iliotibial band.

Press the left thumb into the side of the pelvis and take out the looseness. Then, with your right hand, rotate the thigh inward into medial rotation until you feel the engagement of the ligaments. If you encounter tension as you press in with the left hand, take up the slack, pressing *into* the tension and simultaneously, with the right hand, rotate the leg just a bit more. Hold for a few moments, then clearly disengage.

Now place your left thumb about an inch or so lower (inferior) and a bit more posterior, midway along the tensor fascia lata. You'll be about halfway between the top the pelvis (iliac crest) and the beginning of the thigh (greater trochanter). Repeat the stroke as above. Simultaneously press in with your left thumb and rotate the femur with your right hand. If you find no significant tension when you take out the looseness with the left hand, you don't need to spend much time there.

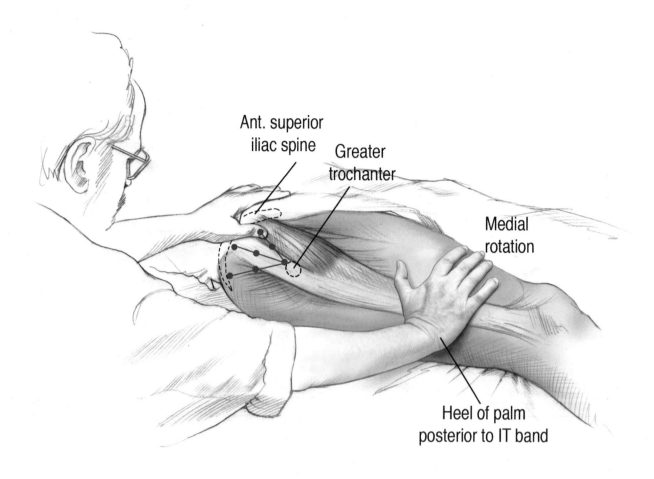

Ant. superior
iliac spine

Greater
trochanter

Medial
rotation

Heel of palm
posterior to IT band

Figure 11. Tensor Fascia Lata, Gluteus Medius, and Gluteus Minimus

Moving on to the next area, press with your left thumb into the soft tissue just above the greater trochanter. Repeat as above. If you find tension, create a fulcrum with the left hand and add inward rotation of the thigh with the right hand to open the hip joint as well as the side of the pelvis.

The rest of the places we'll be working here will be done in a similar manner. The next three areas will be along an imaginary line neatly dividing the front of the body from the back.

Again we begin just beneath the top of the pelvis, then halfway between that point and the top of the greater trochanter, and then just above the top of the greater trochanter. In each case we accompany the pressure into the side of the pelvis with full inward rotation of the thigh, holding somewhat longer when we do find significant tension.

The last three places are perhaps one-half to one inch farther back, and address the posterior fibers of the gluteus medius and gluteus minimus.

Create fulcrums as needed combining inward rotation with direct pressure into the side of the pelvis 1) just beneath the iliac crest; 2) halfway between the crest and the greater trochanter; 3) just above the greater trochanter. Two variants to consider:

- To the inward rotation with the right hand, you may add a little downward (inferior-ward) traction to open the hip joint even more.

- Instead of holding the inward rotation with your right hand, if your intuition says it will be more effective, you can accompany the melting of the tissues in the side of the pelvis with a gentle rocking of the thigh back and forth (inward and outward) in a soothing, flowing rhythm.

Iliotibial Band—"Making Rainbows"

This series of fulcrums was aptly named by our school instructor Cindy Anderson.

Sit on a chair or stool or kneel alongside the client's upper thigh. While performing this stroke you will shift your position so you are always directly facing the area where you are working.

Center yourself and breathe. Touch the tips of your thumbs together with your palms facing away from you, fingers up and thumb pads facing medially. The thumbs together make a curve, a kind of rainbow shape.

Place your curved thumbs beneath the beginning of the thigh, just inferior to the greater trochanter, feel for the tendon that runs down the side of the thigh, the iliotibial band. Now place your thumbs well behind (posterior to) this tendon.

This area of the body can be extraordinarily tender. Be sure to check in periodically with the client to affirm that this feels deeply pleasant and doesn't hurt.

Change the direction of your thumb pads so that they now face anteriorly (toward the sky). Staying behind the tendon and not slipping over it, gently take out the looseness. Then take up the slack, feeling an optimal clarity of contact and gently stretching it. Lift the tendon skyward with your curved thumbs and hold it up. If the client's leg is light and seems to float up too easily or rolls away from you, feel free to use the fingers of both hands to press down lightly on the thigh, stabilize it while you lift the tendon with your thumbs. Where you do sense a fulcrum is appropriate, spend a little extra time, building it—holding the tendon up, stretching it, while letting the client give you the weight of their whole leg.

When you see a working sign or when you sense the fulcrum has been held long enough, clearly disengage. Then create another fulcrum about two inches lower down the side of the thigh. Repeat as above. Depending on the length of the client's leg, you will make contact with five or more places along the side of the thigh. End an inch or so above the knee.

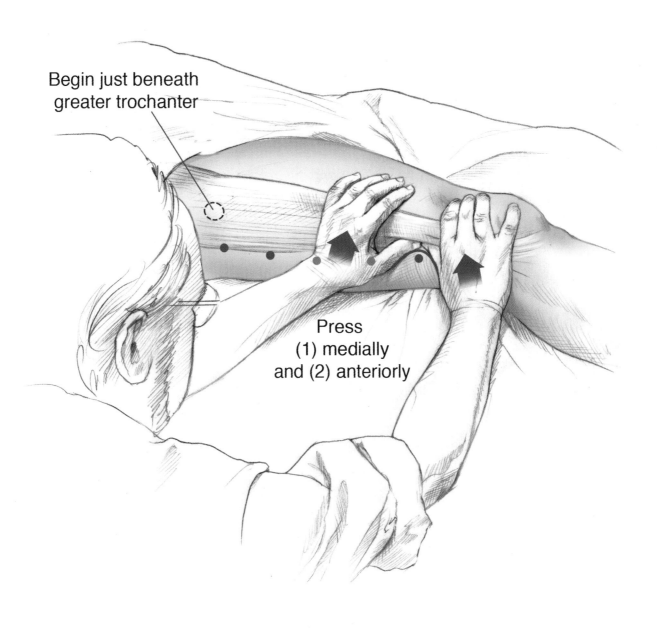

Begin just beneath
greater trochanter

Press
(1) medially
and (2) anteriorly

Figure 12. Iliotibial Band ("Making Rainbows")

Peroneus Longus and Brevis (AKA Fibularis)

This essentially involves "making rainbows" on the side of the lower leg.

Sit or kneel alongside the client's lower leg, facing just below the knee. Place your curved thumbs just posterior to the muscles running down the side of the lower leg, the peroneus longus and brevis (also called the fibularis). These muscles lie on the side of the thinner leg bone, the fibula, and begin about an inch below the knee.

Staying beneath (posterior to) the muscle, gently lift it skyward with your curved thumbs. If the client's leg is very light, feel free to press with your fingers onto the front of the leg to stabilize it. Take out the looseness in the muscle, take up the slack lifting just a bit more and hold your skyward pressure while the client relaxes into it. Hold for three to five seconds; then clearly disengage.

Now place your thumbs about one and a half to two inches lower on the leg and repeat this stroke. Work successive places, each lower on the leg than the last. Depending on the length of the client's leg, you will make four or more strokes. End about an inch above the ankle.

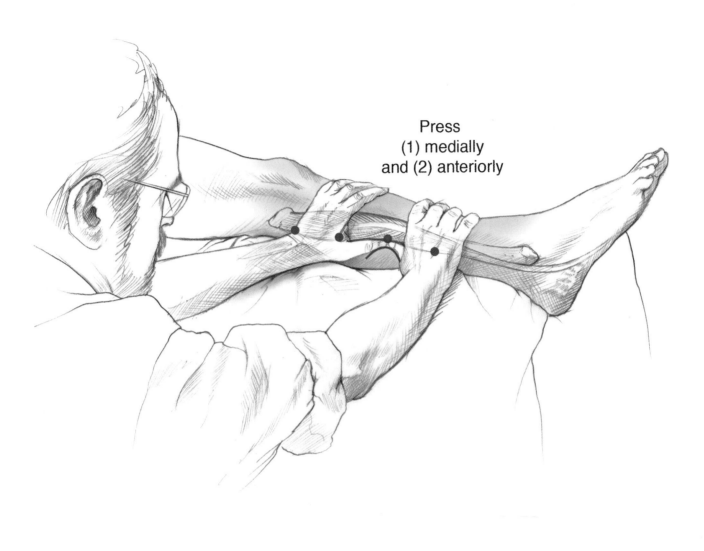

Press
(1) medially
and (2) anteriorly

Figure 13: Peroneus Longus and Brevis (aka Fibularis)

Tibialis Anterior

Stand facing the side of the client at about knee level. If you'll be working on the right leg first, let your legs be about shoulder-width apart with your right foot facing the foot of the table. As you do this stroke you'll be gently bending and leaning into your right leg.

Center yourself, breathing and relaxed. Make a loose fist with your left hand and place it just beneath the knee, next to the shinbone—the tibia. Take out the looseness, pressing into the muscle here, the tibialis anterior. Press slightly downward toward the feet, taking up the slack. Then begin moving inferiorly, slowly following the muscle alongside the tibia down toward the foot.

Maintain your pressure, depth, and direction until you reach the front of the ankle. Then, considerably easing up in pressure, continue the stroke until you reach the instep (where this muscle attaches to the foot).

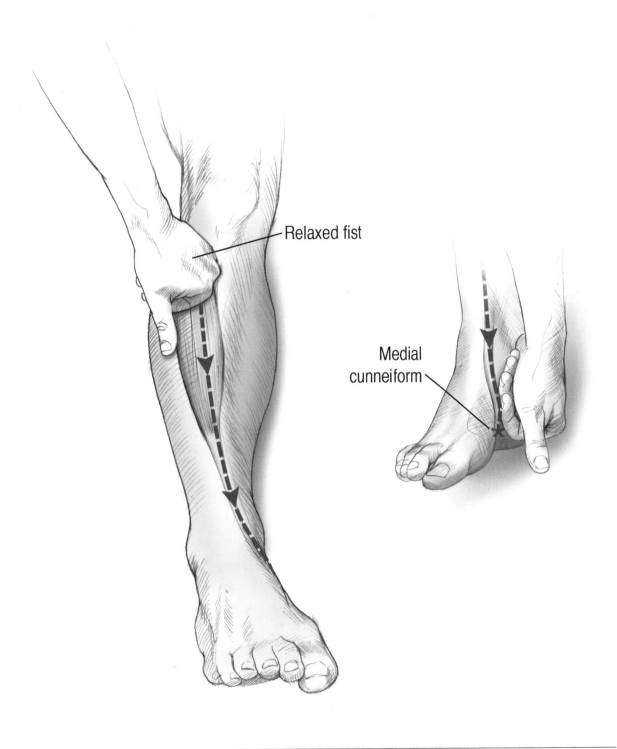

Relaxed fist

Medial
cunneiform

Figure 14. Tibialis Anterior

Half-Moon Vector through the Legs

Most Deep Massage fulcrums are "point of reference" or moving fulcrums. This means we consciously interface with a particular area. Each of these fulcrums may be experienced throughout the whole self, but they originate in interface with a particular muscle, bone, or joint.

There are also "field" fulcrums. These are done with the therapist's attention on the whole body and the entire energy field, not just on a particular area. Through a field fulcrum, we may get a sense of the client's overall level of holding or freedom, mobility or hyper-mobility, heaviness or lightness, and more.

The client's experience is unique in each case. Common effects from this fulcrum include a wonderfully amplified sense of being grounded yet buoyant; an experience of unity, of being whole, not just in parts; sensing a river of energy flowing along one's entire length; a sense of letting go through one's entire being.

Deep Massage works with clearer, stronger force fields than those that may be present. It overrides less well-held fields such as misalignment, joint compression, tension, unsettling emotions, and confusion. The Half-Moon Vector through the Legs has the effect of overriding tensions held within the whole of body, mind, and spirit.

Position yourself comfortably, standing at the foot of the table, with one foot behind the other. Center yourself, breathing, relaxed, and attentive. Place your hands under the feet and ankles of your client.

Let the little finger side of your hand be behind the calcaneus and your fingers under the calcaneal "Achilles" tendon. If the client is noticeably turned out or in, gently lift and bring their legs to a neutral position. This fulcrum is for the whole self, so excessive rotation in the ankle, knees, or hips can diminish access to the whole length of the person.

Take out the looseness by feeling for the precise shape of the calcaneus and its tendon. Form-fit and nestle into that shape with your palm and fingers. Do not press in with your thumbs, just let them rest on the tops or sides of the legs or feet, wherever they naturally fall.

Next, let your body's weight shift slightly back from your front leg to your rear leg and let that shift gently take up the slack from the whole body.

Now add the "Half-Moon." Tuck your pelvis under slightly. This will gently pull on your arms and hands, giving you a slight additional curved traction.

There are two main ways to put in the Half-Moon. During the session feel for which may work best.

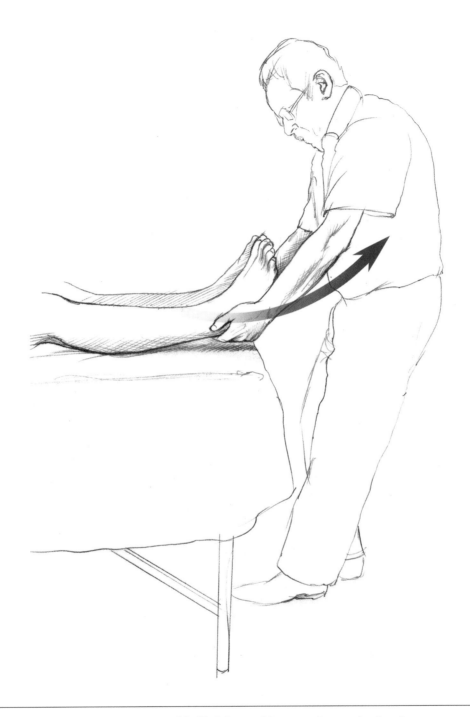

Figure 15. Half-Moon Vector through the Legs

You can, after the firm straight pull ("taking up the slack"), add additional traction and, as you traction, go slightly down, then up, describing a curve, yet you end up holding without your shoulders raised. In this way the Half-Moon's end is just as high as its beginning. Alternatively, after the firm straight pull, you can add additional traction up, both lifting and lengthening.

When you put in the Half-Moon, make sure you do not pull with effort. The point is to clearly engage the client with a gentle curved pull. It is really more a feeling of opening than traction.

After you put in the Half-Moon, go to a witness state. Hold it… hold it… hold it… Allow the client time in which to sink into progressively deeper levels of letting go.

When you sense it has been long enough or when you see a working sign, clearly disengage. Give the client some moments to integrate the experience.

This fulcrum can be repeated at various times during the session. If you start with a Half-Moon through the legs, it gives you initial information and gives the client's structure and energy a reference point for the session. Midway through the session, especially after working on the pelvis, legs, and/or feet, it integrates the work on the lower body and sets the stage for upper body work. At the end of a session, I always finish with a Half-Moon Vector through the Legs. It is grounding; it gives the client a last opportunity to let go of any remaining residual tension in the energy field; and it is a summation for the whole session.

Massage and the Vertical Truth: Graceful Verticality—The Fourth Dimension of Touch

*Two forces rule the universe —
light and gravity.*

— Simone Weil

Our evolution from quadruped to biped is an accomplishment we each still aspire to perfect. How miraculous and risky it is to balance on two limbs! Observe a child taking those first tentative steps, teetering from side to side in the attempt to balance simultaneously the front with the back, the oblique ever-changing planes of locomotion, the coordination of limbs, the positioning, flexing, rotating, and swaying axial body segments. Standing and moving the body forward is a challenging undertaking, fraught with complexity!

As well, in reaching verticality, we expose the most sensitive and vulnerable parts of ourselves—the underbelly and the genitals. We find ourselves precariously balancing on two legs, our undersides exposed as we move over the Earth with a wing and a prayer—and we're supposed to be okay with this!?

The fourth dimension of touch is created by the structural and energetic impact of posture. Posture—how we stand, how we position and carry ourselves along our various paths through our lives, how we grow, is in fact a matter of the deepest feeling and concern.

To understand posture in its fullness, it helps to look at our models for growing up, for how we stand and move literally and figuratively through our time and space. In our society, attaining adulthood is often viewed as a loss. Being an adult stereotypically implies forsaking the joy, the innocence, and the freedom of childhood. Adults often grumble about the scarcity of time and the overabundance of responsibilities.

However, when we move beyond such a conventional view, we may find opportunities to create the life we consciously want. It is possible to love your work, enjoy a contented family life, feel creative and resourceful, and apply yourself to working out your conscious evolution.

It is worth noting that energy, since it is neither created nor destroyed, does not age. Furthermore, with the appropriate care, our physical structure continues to evolve and unfold new possibilities and new levels of health as we learn more about ourselves.

Growing up is our pathway to expand beyond ourselves, to move ever upward and out of our old boundaries and limitations and into a greater understanding of our life and the individual possibilities for our creative expression. It brings with it the opportunity to stand and move in ever greater harmony with our inner and outer nature.

Aldous Huxley described standing in balance structurally with the nature around and within us as "animal grace." With it we align with the great force of gravity and our brilliant structure, which uses the inherent buoyancy of water and the electromechanical arrangements of fascia in harmony with our other systems to ensure our buoyancy and balance within the gravitational field.

Bodywork and the Vertical Energy Flow

Both the biomechanical and the energetic models of posture aim at standing and moving in balance. Western biology, while often not acknowledging energy per se, offers a detailed description of the predominantly vertical orientation of our anatomy. Picture the skeletal, nervous, muscular, cardiovascular, and lymphatic systems. Physics defines "energy" as the capacity for action or "work done." The work of our physiological systems is executed predominantly in the vertical.

Equally remarkable and exciting is that all models for energy flow correlate with this overall direction. Whether we are looking at the model of polarity, the meridians of traditional Chinese medicine, Wilhelm Reich's orgonomy, the chakras, kundalini, ayurveda, or, more recently, Zero Balancing, and Tom Myers' myofascial anatomy trains, all agree that the major currents of energy within us flow vertically.

What implications does this have for growth, defined as living in ever greater harmony with nature, and for touch therapy?

Growth is a process of discovering, and gradually shedding, the physical and emotional tensions that no longer serve us. As we let these tensions go, the freed body lengthens; it ascends. The energy we used just to hold ourselves in a certain position is reduced. We have more energy freely available for our lives. Self-growth is not just a psychological concept. It is literal. We grow a new body, we get bigger, more open inside. We grow the body, mind, and heart that we want.

As we become more easily balanced, a qualitative change of being is experienced. Energy flows more freely through us; we are literally nourished by the vertical energy flow. We feel ourselves balanced by natural forces, not merely by our own will. In balance we feel the washing away of unnecessarily held tensions. In this rigorous sense, vertical alignment is inherently purifying. Verticalizing practices such as yoga, tai chi, martial arts, and other enlightened forms of movement coaching can be fundamental to our further evolution and growth.

For touch therapy, this situation gives us a straightforward ticket to the miraculous. As Rolfing and other verticalizing body therapies have shown, we can lengthen and facilitate new buoyancy for our clients. In releasing the fascia and the interconnected physiological and psychological tensions, we usefully bring healthy boundaries and new possibilities of freedom to light. We facilitate the awareness and release of tensions that normally lie below the client's level of consciousness. As we facilitate this deeper psycho-physical letting go, we help accelerate and balance a growth process. The educative impact of this results in a self-sustaining momentum for further opening and growth.

With less need to siphon off the life force just to "hold" ourselves up, increased energy is available for life. Letting go into gravity and the inherent buoyancy of human structure, clients learn that nature can organize our balance quite well, thank you very much! When balance is experienced as a function of the natural world, we feel more connected to nature, akin to all life. We experience ourselves more deeply as truly being a part of things.

"Gravity is the Therapist"

As energy flows more clearly and strongly through the input of the therapist, the client experiences a literal increase of energetic nourishment. With regard to the aligning effect of gravity, Ida Rolf said, "Gravity is the therapist!" Improved alignment allows everyday energetic and structural tensions to flow out from the aligned system more thoroughly and more quickly, rather than accumulating.

The neutrality of gravity and innate postural grace are freely and equally given to us. If God is indeed everywhere, it is certainly manifest in the unconditional support given to every one of us by gravity and the buoyancy inherent in human structure.

In physics, gravity is considered a weak force. At first thought this may seem unlikely to us — gravity is rather forceful in relation to a ton of bricks! Yet consider that when we jump, with just a few twitches of the gastrocnemius, we rise up off the Earth, successfully albeit temporarily countering the gravitational force of an entire planet! In this sense gravity indeed appears to be relatively weak.

For our purposes gravity can be understood as not so much weak as gentle — mild, not heavy. Gravity is the gentleness of white snow falling without wind. As touch therapists we work with the gentleness of the gravitational field rather than with muscular force.

In practice, when we balance and lean in toward our clients using gravity, we are working on them using the energy of an entire planet. If we are out of balance and pushing into the body with muscular effort, we are constrained to the limited and conditioned efforts of a single individual.

Not coincidentally, working with gravity rather than with muscular force can extend our longevity as therapists. Using gravity is much easier! In utilizing the natural buoyancy of our structure to connect our clients to the abundance and the power of gravity, we also expand the experience of our clients. We utilize gravity as a nutritive force.

The concept of the nurturing Earth is ultimately scientific, not just sentimental. Relevant here is the space program discovery that astronauts in zero gravity not only lose muscle and bone mass but also experience a dramatic decrease of red blood cell production in the marrow of their bones! Gravity is nourishment indeed!

The Electricity of Touch

The predominant direction of energy flowing through us is vertical. When we forget to align ourselves consciously and depart from the gracefully vertical, we in effect compromise this energy flow. Hunched over or locked into an overly fixed posture, we literally unplug ourselves from the main energy circuit available to us. Giving (or receiving) a massage when out of vertical alignment doesn't feel quite right.

The corollary of course is terrifically exciting. The more gracefully vertical we are, the more energy there is in our work — the more we "plug" ourselves into the vertical energy flow, our cosmic "light socket."

Touch emanating from enhanced verticality is experienced as having a higher voltage. It participates in the energetic connection of heaven and earth, like lightning — the vertical energy flow made dramatically visible. Experiment with your clients and ask how they experience touch from a therapist with a hunched-over posture versus touch connected to a graceful verticality. Even lying prone with eyes closed, most clients can tell whether or not the therapist is grounded.

Hyper-extended knees will diminish the energy flow by locking it up instead of conducting it. Similarly there's a sense of heaviness, a lack of heavenly connection, when the therapist hunches over and works with a curved spine and medially rotated shoulders — a position that's excessively earthbound.

In gracefully vertical movement and bodywork we easily harness a greater quantity of force by working with the natural energy of gravity and the anti-gravitational forces of our body as we move. Empowered bodywork replaces effort, as much as possible, with balance. When we do this, there is as well a dramatically higher *quality* of energy.

When we are balanced, the force from which we draw runs through the body but is not *of* it. Using gravity and the natural lightness of our buoyancy, we drop the brute force of will, the pushing energetic quality of muscular effort. Our touch acquires a heavenly aspect. Being part animal, part angel, balanced human touch brings in a literally angelic quality while maintaining our connection with the earth. The electricity of touch clearly establishes the connection and the necessary polarities of the angelic and the earthly.

Lightness

Commonly after a bodywork session a client stands up and says, "I feel lighter!" During the hour the person has not actually lost weight, so how do they feel lighter?

The sensation of weight is not a function of mass. The sensation of weight arises largely from tension. It is the extent to which we are tense that determines how heavy we feel. We feel lighter as our tension drops away.

Earlier we described how fascia is thixotrophic, meaning it acquires greater fluidity with greater levels of activity within it. Thus with chronic tension, with diminished freedom, we become quite literally more solid.

Andrew Taylor Still stated, "Movement is health." He formulated the Law of the Artery, postulating that the body contains all the healing substances it needs. It is the therapist's job to facilitate getting them to where they can be used.

Because we are mostly water, it is largely the free flow of water within us that is healing. The dissolution of heaviness and the restoration of lightness result from the free flow of water. Our therapy uses the enlightening power of touch to facilitate this freedom.

The human world is often in danger of becoming too solid. Our upbringing, our education, our culture, and the ways we tend to think and live can make the world seem resistant to change, opaque, heavy. It is important for us to share and cultivate compassion for this feeling of weightiness in living. Gravity may be the therapist, but in some senses gravity is also the problem. What can we do with the sense of spiritual heaviness, the perception of the world as too solid and beyond change?

Science helps us out here. We know that open space is predominantly what there is. All matter is dissolved and flowing within open seas of energy. I once was working on a radiologist. He was talking about how excited he and others in his field were with all the new things they were seeing thanks to magnetic resonance imaging. I asked him, "What are you seeing?" He said, kind of surprised, "Mostly we don't know what it is!" Surprised, too, I asked, "What do you think it is?" "We think," he said, "it's water."

The writer Italo Calvino said, "Knowledge of the world means dissolving the solidity of the world." We are now seeing the solidity of the body dissolved as we develop the ability to look more deeply. As bodyworkers, we have a deep intuitive loyalty to energy as well as structure. The experience of energy dissolves the solidity of the world.

As we work in alignment with the vertical energy flows, we ourselves are literally more fluid, in effect, lighter, because in seeking balance we have let go of unnecessary tension. As we've discovered, when we are in balance with nature, we become the conduit for a greater quality and quantity of energy. Clients experience an enhanced energy flow when touched by a therapist who embodies energetic and structural balance. The solidity of their being eases and they experience more lightness, more openness to change.

Therapy helps to restore the flow within form. As we feel energy flow within us, we experience greater lightness. We experience moments of illumination. As many of us have observed in our practice, our work is often a source of dramatic illumination for body, mind, and spirit. Sudden insights, emotional breakthroughs, dramatic shifts of self-image, or accelerations to new levels of spiritual connectedness commonly accompany the most successful moments of our sessions.

Perhaps the inner light turned on by graceful human touch is the bodily-felt answer to the question: What does it feel like to live an unforced life? After all, clients often seek bodywork when life has become too difficult. Touch therapy, by harnessing the vertical energy flow, dissolves our illusion of the world's solidity. We see the light, not just opacity. We are open to change. We don't need to force it. The goal of health care is true ease in this highest of senses, not merely the absence of dis-ease. In structural and energetic balance, we have a bodily felt experience of peace on earth.

May this experience resonate throughout our life and our world!

Stand By Me

It is terrifying, joyous, maddening, inspiring, sad, and mundane to live our lives. What is more, the emotional complexities of participating in the human community can be overwhelming.

In 1962 Ben E. King recorded the song, "Stand by Me." In his refrain, he reminds us that the courage of companionship will see us through the moments of darkness in our lives.

It seems that the most we can do—and in some ways all we can do—is to truly stand by one another. We can stand up on our own and we stand by our clients. We stand by them in their attempts to soar, with their wings and with their prayers, through this incredible world. Touching them, from a balanced place, we hope to facilitate their evolution and our own—this growing up of humanity.

As touch professionals and as individuals who value touch, may we stand by one another in fullest appreciation of this extraordinary opportunity.

The Front Torso—Anatomy, Energy, and Fulcrums

As noted in Chapter 7, The Back, in a truly three-dimensional experience of oneself, there is no front and no back as such. There is an elongated cylinder that is the torso. Within that unity there are distinctions to be made, many of them bound up with our psycho-emotional identity.

To start, the front of the cylinder feels and looks different than the back. Uniquely, the front features three intimate landmarks—the navel and the nipples—as well as a large and vulnerable personal area, the belly. Most everywhere else, bones protect and surround our vital organs: the ribs around the lungs and heart, the cranium around the brain, the vertebrae around the spinal cord.

In four-legged animals the belly is not nearly as exposed. With the human belly, nature made a bold exception. Evolution finds us upright, the belly in the forefront,

like a previously downturned face suddenly turned upward. How remarkable is this opportunity to meet each other head-on, face-to-face, and belly-to-belly! Designed originally to be the least exposed, bellies now hang out (often literally) front and center for all to see. The craving for a six-pack or a last bite of brownie further complicates our inordinate preoccupation with belly size and shape.

Above the belly lies the chest, with its own host of existential meanings. Such strong associations and virtues accompany this part of our anatomy—the manly chest, the feminine breasts, the brave heart, the milk of human kindness.

As therapists we cannot fail to consider that the front thorax may equally mirror early emotional challenges in life. A concave or deflated chest may reflect the weight of defeat or disappointment. The rigidly convex or chronically inflated chest may reflect the unhealed wounds of trauma, with the person valiantly determined to hold themselves erect, maintaining their pride by never fully exhaling.

It is not obvious at first, but much of the structural and muscular life of the torso is ultimately connected to the movements and emotions expressed by the shoulder girdle, arms, and hands. The first layer of the posterior torso is a shoulder girdle muscle, the latissimus dorsi, which begins on the pelvis and sacrum and forms the back wall of the armpit, finally attaching to the anterior humerus.

Similarly the pectoralis major, the front muscle of the chest, interdigitates or interweaves with the main belly muscle, the rectus abdominis, which anchors on the pubic bone of the pelvis. Lift your arms high overhead and you will feel the stretch of your front torso all the way down through your waist to the pelvis.

Anatomy Review

The spine lies at the center of the torso like the core running through the center of an apple. Recall that at the front of the spine are the thick skeletal bodies of the vertebrae separated by the mostly fluid intervertebral discs. Between the vertebral bodies and the spinous processes there is a ring, an open canal through which the spinal nerves and cerebrospinal fluid flow.

A revelation for me was a conversation I once had with a radiologist. I asked, of all the amazing things he had seen, what stood out in his memory as the most miraculous?

He said it was seeing a living spinal cord for the first time. I was surprised, as I had seen spinal cords only after dissection. They looked like a bunch of yellowish wires hanging down, like tentacles of a dead jellyfish.

I asked him what he meant. He said, "It looks like it's dancing to the Rolling Stones." He said in a living person the spinal cord is constantly and rhythmically moving.

He noted that the spinal cord is not "nailed down" anywhere along its length, unlike the wiring in our houses, which is carefully secured, as otherwise the wires would arc as electricity passes through them. In our anatomical makeup the electricity that passes along the length of the spinal cord, as it freely floats in the cerebrospinal fluid, causes the spinal cord to rhythmically undulate!

This image reminded me of something fundamental that we often forget in studying anatomy. The body is always moving inside! Anatomy books portray everything two-dimensionally and statically. Such misperceptions seriously compromise most people's image of the body.

Remember that each of us internally is a flowing, complex, moving body of water. Our living oceans have rhythmic currents, undulating substances, and fluid tissues. As a therapist, when you touch a body remember that you are touching something that is in flowing motion, just as you yourself are in motion everywhere within yourself. When we do bodywork, we are waves touching waves, two currents coming into relation with one another.

The belly contains more organs than anywhere else in the body and yet it gets little respect. Here are found the stomach, spleen, pancreas, liver, small intestine, large intestine, and gallbladder. Nowhere else in the body do we find such an incredible level of organ diversity. As we work in the abdominal area, let us remember to give this compelling and vital anatomical landscape full acknowledgement for its amazing and life-enhancing contributions to our being.

All the stars make waves everywhere inside of you.

Rectus Abdominis

I recommend asking your client before the session begins if they are fine with you working on their belly. Since it's a more vulnerable and possibly more defended area, some people prefer it not be included. However, most will be fine, especially if we respectfully ask their permission and then work the area with clarity and care.

Working with the rectus abdominis can lead to enormous psychological and physical benefit. So central is it to our being that it is arguably the most important muscle we can work on. (However, I say that about all the muscles! They're like children—it's good to love and respect each one on an individual basis.)

The most serious and common structural distortion we see through the torso is forward flexion. That compromises our posture, compresses our organs, and forces the back to constantly strain to overcome the effects of gravity pulling us forward and down.

Some major gains of working here are to give dramatic relief from back tension, to restore uprightness, and to decompress the organs and spine. With realignment of the back, the neck and head follow it up. Rectus abdominis work also helps restore the head to its rightful position above the torso, rather than hanging out in front of it.

In addition, the rectus abdominis is interwoven with fibers from the other abdominal muscles that go around the entire waist. Therefore, the healthy effects of working here commonly radiate around to the back. Indeed, when a client's tense back muscles are too sensitive to be touched, fulcrums into the rectus abdominis can give dramatic relief of the spasm without ever having to touch the back!

Ideally, the rectus abdominis is stretched with every full inhalation. When it's shortened or tensed, this limits the fullness of the breath. With diminished breath, there is diminished cellular respiration, which then compromises functioning throughout the entire organism.

Energetically, the rectus abdominis is linked to a whole world of feeling and sensation—intuition, deep feelings, courage, fortitude, freedom of breath, the digestion and assimilation of experiences, even an uplifted heart. Biologists now recognize the belly region as home to the "second" brain, called the "enteric" nervous system. This vast and semi-independent community of nerves is responsible for all the actions and interactions of our visceral organs.

Soothing the enteric nervous system and freeing tension in the belly will help balance and optimize the signals these nerves send to the stomach, spleen, pancreas, bladder, small and large intestines, liver, and gallbladder.

With this vast array of effects, it is not surprising that Asian cultures have pointedly identified this area, especially the lower abdomen, as the center of our whole being. Located in the precise center of gravity, the *hara* in Japanese, or *dan tien* in Chinese, is an area approximately two inches in front of the second sacral segment. Traditionally and energetically, the *hara* is regarded as the emotional and physical center of the body from which our energy radiates in all directions just like a sun.

A reminder on boundaries: the rectus abdominis, through its attachments to the pelvis and upper ribs, extends as high as nipple level with fascial continuity up to the base of the neck. It spans and touches on a number of private areas.

Before the session, ask for permission to work in this area. During the work session, be sensitive to the client's sense of boundaries and check in as needed, being extremely clear where you are going and why.

Center yourself as you begin. Stand at pelvis level facing up toward the torso at about 45°. Let's assume we are starting with the client's right side, with the belly undraped.

Place the whole of your right palm on the lower belly. The heel of the hand is just above the side of the pelvis, palm and fingers aiming approximately at the area a few inches beneath the navel. Let the warmth of the whole hand resting here provide reassurance in this sensitive area.

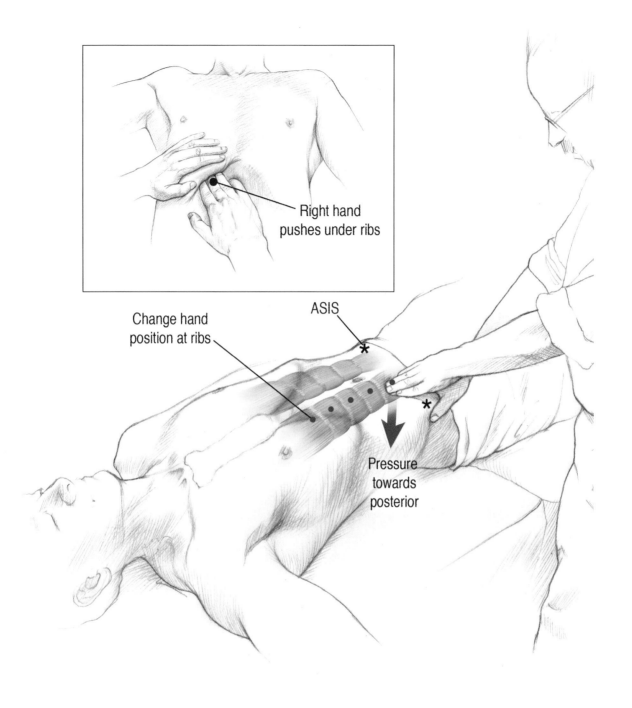

Right hand
pushes under ribs

Change hand
position at ribs

ASIS
*

*

Pressure
towards
posterior

Figure 16. Rectus Abdominis

You will be starting this fulcrum working into the thickest part of the belly of the rectus abdominis muscle, about one inch lateral to the body's midline.

Place your left palm on top of your right hand. Gently press the finger pads of the left hand onto those of the right, and take out the looseness with direct pressure into the rectus abdominis. The direction is posterior, i.e. toward the table surface.

Take a moment to further free your own breath. Then gently relax your knees just a little, using this relaxation to rest just a bit further into the belly of the rectus abdominis, taking up the slack. The client should feel NO discomfort. Now, not necessarily pressing in further but just resting, allow the client to breathe and to relax any tension held at this level in the rectus abdominis. Even if you find no tension, do rest in for the duration of one breath.

Better to err on the conservative side with shorter fulcrums, rather than overworking—each fulcrum here will usually be three to five seconds. Have faith in the cumulative effect of successive points and the healing impact of yourself working with deep relaxation, giving the client nonverbal permission to rest, relax, and heal from inside out.

Now clearly disengage, gently lifting off on the client's inhale. Pause. Then start approximately an inch and a half higher and, following the same steps as above, do a fulcrum into the rectus abdominis at this next level up.

The keys to comfort while working here are 1) the overall warmth of contacting the belly with your whole palm; 2) the specificity of contacting the rectus abdominis in the thickest part of its belly, halfway between the midline and its lateral border; 3) working only as deeply as is comfortable for your client—contact here is much more important than depth.

Repeat these steps in successively higher places up the abdomen, each time clearly disengaging, pausing and re-engaging an inch-and-a-half or so higher. Usually I will do five fulcrums and perhaps more depending on the length of the client's waist.

For the last fulcrum into the belly (Figure 16, insert), just beneath the ribcage let your upper hand gently create more looseness, tractioning ribs seven and eight down. Then with your right hand, you can more comfortably work beneath their ribs, melting in toward the right shoulder.

The next phase of work is with the rectus abdominis and its fascia. We'll first describe working on a man and then revisit boundary issues of men and women.

When we have finished the fulcrums into the abdominal part of this muscle, we shift to working with its tendons and the fasciae with which they interweave. These fibers extend up the body of the sternum and medial costal cartilages to the fifth rib, the level of the nipples—quite high up!

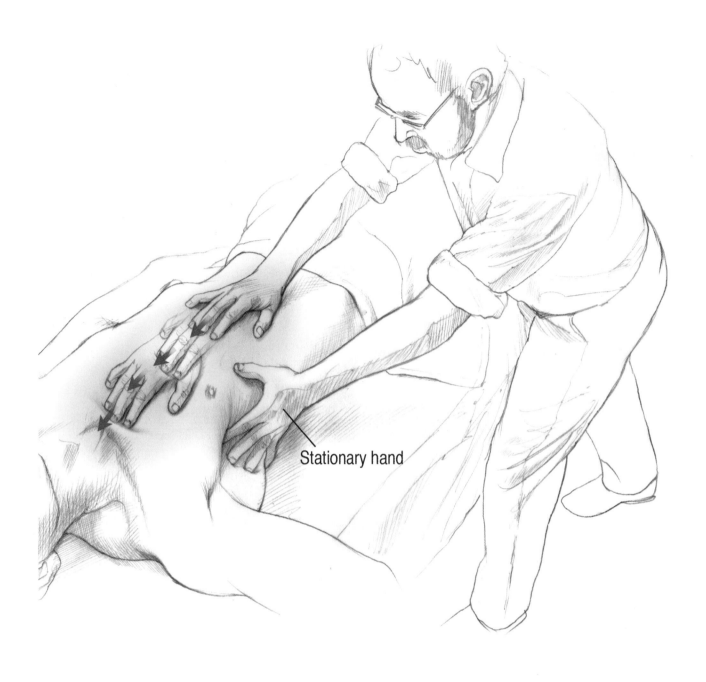

Stationary hand

Figure **17.** Rectus Abdominis/Pectorialis Major—Tendons

Then the fascia interdigitates with that of the pectoralis major and, with it, extends up to the undersurface of the clavicle, near its attachment to the sternum.

First, change your body position. The point of working here is explicitly to lift up the front of the ribcage.

For a male patient you can now undrape the chest.

Position your feet even further down the table (about at the level of the knees) so that as you lean into this fulcrum you will be more in the horizontal plane.

Place your right palm with fingers gently curved and in between the costal cartilages 7-8. You are just lateral to the xiphoid process, which is at the bottom of the sternum. For this entire sliding fulcrum, you must err on the side of being overly medial rather than lateral (especially with women).

Place your left palm, fingers naturally spread, along the side of the ribcage. This hand will be gently tractioning the whole ribcage upward, whilst the right hand, where your primary interface is, will be stretching the fascia of the rectus abdominis and pectoralis major up the sternum and medial costal cartilages.

Your whole right hand is virtually flat, heel resting gently on the upper abdomen and finger pads on the lower cartilages and sternum. Take out the looseness by gently sinking in between the costal cartilage, curving your fingers a little. Simultaneously take out the looseness by gently yet clearly pressing into the ribcage with your left palm.

Now take up the slack with both hands. Your left hand adds upward traction to the ribcage with your right hand adding a vector of stretch to the rectus tendons toward the head. Add additional vectors, particularly with the right hand, where your primary focus lies. Begin a slow, deep effleurage (myofascial traction) up the front of the sternum and medial costal cartilages. Your main interface is between your finger pads and the musculoskeletal landscape you're traveling through.

Continue to ascend slowly. As you sustain this slow-moving fulcrum, feel not only the stretching of the rectus and pectoral tendons but also the ribs lifting, the spaces between them opening up, and the client's breathing opening things from inside out.

Monitor for working signs and overall relaxation, and use these to inform the rhythm of your movement.

Your left hand remains mostly stationary, encouraging a wonderful uplifting sensation by tractioning the ribcage upward (headward). You may choose to position the left hand higher at some point so the client feels clearly addressed at more or less the same level by both hands.

Sustain this long moving fulcrum until the fingers of the right hand contact the undersurface of the clavicle just near its sternal end. Hold for a moment. This point is given a wonderful name in Chinese medicine; it is the very last point on the kidney meridian, translated as "Elegant Mansion."

Now clearly disengage. Pause. Give the client time to integrate the experience and enjoy their new length, the greater room for breath, the deep relief of tension held in the belly and heart areas.

Repeat these steps on the left side, switching which hands are working. As on the right, you will do point of reference fulcrums as needed into the belly of the rectus abdominis, and then a long moving fulcrum to the rectus and its associated fasciae and ribs above the belly up as far as the undersurface of the clavicle near the sternum.

It is important to note that when working the rectus abdominis of a female patient this area remains draped. Additionally, my preference here is first to make sure I have permission, before the session begins, to work in the area of the sternum.

For the clearest draping, hold a pillowcase with the longer length between your hands. Hold the right upper corner with your right hand and the left lower corner with your left hand. Lift the left lower corner up to the right upper corner. This will give you a drape with the folded pillowcase shaped into two triangles. Place the folded pillowcase over the sheet in a position so that, when you pull the sheet down, the folded pillowcase clearly drapes the breasts.

Stabilize the pillowcase at its top, along the clavicles, then pull the sheet down to the level of the lower ribcage.

For a female patient, you can freely work up the sternum and medial costal cartilages with one important difference. With a woman (if working on the right side) let your right hand work up to the level of the fifth rib. Then disengage the right hand and with your left hand fingers pointing down, coming from above the drape, pull up from ribs 5-3 with the left hand. Finally, for the last inch or so, work up again with the right hand (which is easier on the wrist).

The Role of the Heart in Bodywork—
The Fifth Dimension of Touch

In writing about the role of the heart in massage and bodywork, at first there seems to be little to say, but much to feel and do. The heart appears to simply call for us to truly care, and to act in an appropriate and compassionate manner with regard to our clients. I am daunted to speak of or for the heart. It is most eloquent on its own terms. But please accept, ideally as nourishment for our hearts, the following reflections.

Recall that touch, as we are exploring it, reveals itself to be multi-dimensional. Resting your hand on a client's body creates a one-dimensional point of contact between you and your client. The movement of your strokes creates the heightened experience of two-dimensional planes of being. Breathing creates the sense of volume and three-dimensionality. Your vertical posture harnesses the fourth dimension of touch, the energy flowing vertically through each of us.

Massage clients sometimes comment on receiving touch that is accomplished with skill and integrity with regard to the above four dimensions, but which may not be very heartfelt. Thus it is here, beginning with the heart, that the fifth dimension of touch, the power of love, comes to play an essential role in our work. Health-care cannot take place without care in our hearts.

The Living Landscape of the Heart

The heart region is as majestic in its structure as it is in its energy. Anteriorly lies the sternum, the longest part of which is called the gladiolus, from the Latin word for wild iris and for sword. Connecting the sternum and/or the vertebrae are our ribs.

In Western anatomy only the lower two of our twenty-four ribs are called "floating." However, in real life we notice an important truth about the ribs in a freed body: they rise and fall ever on the wings of breath. All our ribs should be thought of as "floating" ribs. The perpetual motion of this area is embodied even in the rhythmic undulation of the spinal nerves.

The dance of life is continuous in every part of us, not the least in our very core. This core movement is of course in concert with the rhythmic movement of other key organs in this region—the beating of the heart, the pulsing of blood vessels, and the expansion and contraction of pulmonary respiration.

The lower boundary of this region is the diaphragm. Significantly, the pericardium—the fascial sheathing of the heart—arises from the superior surface of the diaphragm. We can envision the fascial connection of the beating heart and the breath.

The lungs in turn surround the heart, making this region an unparalleled rhythmic and structural nexus as the lungs and heart respond to ever-changing life needs as interpreted by the neuroendocrine system.

Behind and above the heart lies the trapezius, one of our major musculo-energetic shock absorbers. More internally are found other shoulder girdle and back muscles. When the emotional weight of life becomes too great to bear, these may suffer from deeper structural and energetic impingements. In front of the heart is stationed the pectoralis major, which may express the desire to reach out and touch or the desire to strike or to push away.

Protection and Intimacy

The heart plays a pivotal role in the inner movement between defense and intimacy. When we perceive a threat, either from without or within, we often tense up the muscles around the heart as if to form a shield. Interestingly, Chinese medicine identifies this function as its own organ, separate from the heart, called the "pericardium" or "heart protector."

Each of us must develop a healthy capacity to protect the heart. However, as we have felt with so many clients, self-protection can become a chronic disadvantage. We can lock in tensions around our hearts and grow to inhabit defensive postures and attitudes. Posturally, we may fixate our hidden hearts with forward flexion of the spine or an armored rigid shielding. Our nervous system may constantly replay traumatic challenges from childhood long after we have become, at least outwardly, adults.

Our immune system is key to the body's natural inner defenses. Perhaps it is no accident that nature has placed next to the heart one of the major members of the immune system—the thymus gland. The thymus gland aids and hosts the potentiation of B-cells, generated in the bone marrow. B-cells become any of several categories of T-cells, which are primary players in maintaining health through their role in identifying, guarding, and eliminating disease-causing cells and molecules. Their role, as is true of the immune system in general, is to distinguish between self and non-self substances and to defend us against the non-self. Thus we see another way in which the heart region, archetypically, is involved in physiological defense.

When habitually defended, however, we may defend even against vital parts of our selves. We learn to disown or abhor certain "negative" feelings—anger, fear, envy, grief. We learn to treat them as if they were non-self substances, chronically rejecting certain feelings as surely as we might a pathogen or implanted organ. No wonder that psychotherapist Wilhelm Reich claimed that cancer was a result of living in a habitually defended manner.

We can well imagine the physiological consequences of chronically defending against vital parts of ourselves. A crucial role of the therapist becomes to restore the structural and energetic health of the heart area. With our own hearts open we can facilitate the safe and timely letting go of physical and psychic injuries against which we have maintained obsolete and compromising levels of defense. The heart's opening moves us out of hyper-immunity, out of the chronically defended life, into community and the enhanced capacity for intimacy with ourselves and others.

Therapeutic Bravery

At first thought it would seem to take little bravery to be a massage therapist. Courage is not a word one would ordinarily associate with massage or bodywork. Yet beneath the surface of our work, bravery lives in our hearts as much as does compassion.

There are two distinct aspects of compassion. The first, and the most common, is niceness. Being nice involves expressing our sweeter impulses and excluding all others. Bodywork, as with many healing professions, is afflicted with an abundance of niceness. The problem is, since being nice involves the active repression of all other impulses and feelings, it is itself essentially repressive. There's even something a little sneaky about it, in that niceness aims to disarm the outside world, while allowing all the less savory aspects of ourselves to remain in hiding.

Bodywork can be extremely frustrating. Let it be said! Sometimes the resistance of clients to change drives me crazy. Sometimes I'm frustrated by events in my own life that are totally remote from the therapy — car trouble, time crunches, fluctuating self-esteem, dietary indiscretions.

Allowing all our feelings as well as all our movements, thoughts, and spiritual attitudes means that we adopt radical compassion as our therapeutic stance. I say radical because inherent in this is the commitment to receiving all our experiences with kindness. "Kindness" here is used literally in its relationship to what is kindred. All our feelings — anger, joy, fear, love, grief — are equally valid and relevant parts of us.

From this stance comes bravery — because it takes courage to walk through this field, in which we commit to accepting all of ourselves and all of our clients. It requires bravery not just in the sense of courage of the heart, but also in the sense emerging from the Latin origin, *bravo*, meaning bold, wild, savage.

Bravery is the second and more radical aspect of compassion. Wildness is necessary to be a therapist. Wildness enables us to fully enter into and compassionately accept all of what is real.

When we commit ourselves to embodying radical compassion, we accept that we will work with hearts wide open to everything there is. This is perhaps the bravest, the wildest thing we can do.

In wildness is the preservation of the world.

— Henry David Thoreau

The Energetic Geography of the Heart

Physics posits a universe of energy and structure. Objects can be conceived as waveforms or as organized particles. The denser the matter, the denser the energy flow, the more the vibrations contained.

Anatomically, the skeletal system may be regarded as the conveyor of the most concentrated energy, as it is composed of the densest matter in the body. Much as the water of a river within its meandering banks, or as air currents in fluctuating weather patterns, we can visualize energy swirling and eddying in the irregular and curving forms of living bones. As the spinal curves reverse from lordotic (inward) to kyphotic (outward), we can observe energy whorls along the vertical column of the body. These may be viewed as corresponding to the chakras, the energy centers of yogic anatomy. Each energy center functions both structurally and energetically.

Let us consider the nature of the heart region in its relation to other centers in the body. Almost immediately our examination reveals a striking fact: over half the length of the spine is devoted to the region of the heart! Whereas the root chakra, for instance, primarily corresponds to the region of the coccyx, and the second chakra to the region of the sacrum, the region of the heart has correspondence with all twelve large thoracic vertebrae. Given its

variety of energetic states, one fundamental fact emerges: the heart region is the largest energetic and structural domain in the human body.

By devoting so much space to the heart center, nature has allowed it to play the largest role of all in our lives. Whereas our culture appears to be head-centered, human biology remains unalterably heart-centered. If spaciousness is indeed the essential nature, it is no surprise that this region is our emotional center, home to the vast array of our worldly feelings. Bravery resides in the heart because, literally and figuratively, therein is the greatest capacity. Here flutter the wings of breath and the pulsating rhythm of our beating heart. Here reside the shield and the sword and the wild iris. Here are the floating ribs, the undulating intelligence of the spine and the heart's articulation through the free expression of ribs, shoulder girdle, arms, and hands.

Massage and the Imagery of the Heart

In an earlier chapter, we looked at the vertical energy flow and its relevance to life and to massage. Energy flows vertically through us because our anatomic and physiologic processes mostly happen in the vertical. In this sense we may say that the major direction of energy flow is between heaven and earth. As it flows, at each level of our selves, this swirling energy contributes

something unique to our lives. Below the heart are the three lower chakras. From the first, we derive stability and grounding; from the second, sexuality, life force, and exhilaration; and from the third, our stamina, the power for our individual life.

With our arrival at the fourth chakra, the spirit of the heart, something new occurs.

For the first time, we relate expansively to the world outside us; we are no longer exclusively self-centered. Basic confidence, having come from positively experiencing our balance, our sexuality, and our power, allows us to grow further. We want to partake in what is to be done, and to share who we are, not just for our own sake, but because, with our sense of self somewhat assured, we have more than enough energy to support others as well. Our cup runneth over.

Our energy flows into the spacious area of the heart like a spring into a lake. Just as we have been nourished and formed through our early years, we now have the natural inclination to sustain and support the vast world spread out around us. As we flow into the heart chakra, we naturally feel gratitude for the gift of life. We connect with the sense that life comes not from ourselves, but flows abundantly through us.

Love is the emanation of our gratitude. It naturally flows out through our work, helping to shape the world. Recall the words of Pablo Neruda: "Hands make the world each day."

The energy of the heart region, through the intermediary of the ribs, shoulders, arms, and hands, flows both vertically and the horizontally. Esoterically, the symbolic and archetypal shape of a cross gives us the intersection of horizontal and vertical axes at precisely the level of the human heart.

Here is the living crossroads in each of us, where we are given the opportunity to balance the vertical energy supporting us and the horizontal flow of energy that connects us. In ideal balance, through our hearts, we experience connection with the world of Mother Earth, with the spirit, as well as our kinship with all life around us.

Above the heart are three more chakras: the throat chakra, entryway for breath and its transmutation into the expression of individual truth; the forehead or "third eye" through which we can see the truth; and the crown chakra, through which we connect with the truth beyond ourselves.

Below the heart are three centers for power, excitement, and grounding. With three chakras above the heart and three below it, this places the heart at our precise energetic center. The energetic centrality of the heart, as a living fulcrum between our higher and lower selves, is expressed beautifully and profoundly in an ancient Chinese medical classic: "Heaven and Earth meet in the Heart. It is their destiny and place of rendezvous."

The Myth of Back Pain

These discussions encourage us to take a new look at what we call "back pain." With a deeper understanding of inappropriate levels of self-defense or socially enforced restrictions on self-awareness, we can virtually feel the origin of much so called "back" pain. When we restrict the flow of movement in the heart region or the lumbar or sacral areas, pain eventually ensues. Back pain may originate in the heart region because our first line of defense is often restricted breathing and tensing around the heart.

In this way of perception we see back pain as a malady impeding the free inflow and outflow of spirit. With the exception of acute physical trauma, pain in this region does not originate in the muscles or ligaments. It originates in the mixed messages we send the heart and pelvis, in restricting breathing, the resulting excessive fixations of ribs and vertebrae, and the restricted movement and energy flow through our upper and lower limbs.

"Back pain" is a defended name for what actually is going on here, one that hides more than it reveals. It takes just a moment's pause and a breath to feel that much of back pain is a result of structurally and energetically restricted range of motion in the realm of the heart. To address it we need to be centered, to be brave, and to open up to all of our self and all of our client.

Through this region our touch acquires the compassion we need, encouraging the client's neuroendocrine system to feel safe and let go of unnecessary tension. Then, above all, we need to free the ribs whose movement is essential for the influx and outflow of spirit.

Once the ribs are free, we can use breath and bodywork to re-float the clavicles and the scapulae. Through them we can regain freedom of the heart, reaching out for our heart's desires through the arms and hands. Through them we can restore the sternum's crystalline role in the fostering of courage.

We may also see each rib, as we free it, acting like a fulcrum on the vertebrae themselves, restoring flexibility, length, and movement to the spine. With more freedom to our very core, energy flows more freely vertically as well as horizontally through the body, sustaining us at a higher level and amplifying our connection through all of our being to Earth below and to Heaven above. For chronic back pain, fulfilling our hearts' dreams may be a most profound and welcome remedy.

Our Further Evolution

Our pain points in the direction of our growing edge, our further evolution. Humanity itself is at a crossroads. Holistic health calls for an ever deepening commitment to a more conscious connection to all of ourselves, to one another, to the nature around us, and to the force that gives us life.

How can we overcome our defensive barriers to one another and our resistance to change? The heart, being the crossroads for the vertical and horizontal energy flow, continuously poses for us this evolutionary question. It is from our living crossroads that we must answer. It is from this vantage that we make the world anew each day.

We bear conscious witness to a central miracle in our lives—the human heart as the fertile meeting place of Heaven and Earth. This union of Heaven and Earth manifests our love, and from it the act of touch through the horizontality of shoulders, arms, and hands. When we touch, with the awareness of the structural and energetic spaciousness of the heart, love emanates. When we touch with gratitude and with bravery, when we allow and accept without judgment or comparison, we open into a space much larger than ourselves. Heaven and Earth reach harmony when we touch with the awareness that "love makes the world go 'round."

More deeply, it is not even with our hands that we touch. The desire, the energy, and the inspiration to touch truly originates in our hearts.

In massage therapy we restore the alignment of body, mind, and spirit through the miracle of touching heart-to-heart.

The best and most beautiful things in the world cannot be seen, nor touched... but are felt in the heart.

— Helen Keller

Shoulders, Arms, and Hands— Anatomy, Energy, and Fulcrums

These arms of mine.
And if you would let them hold you
Oh, how grateful I will be.
These arms of mine…
— Otis Redding

In Chinese medicine, the heart expresses itself through the shoulders, arms, and hands. Clearly the upper limb and its girdle have a dynamic role in life, for we take action through this area. We get things we want. We reach out to eat, to embrace, and to accomplish essential tasks at work and at home.

We also enact self-expression. The shoulders, arms, and hands have linguistic as well as gestural functions. We move them almost as parts of speech. Their peaceful, flowing, or forceful movements reveal with connotative clarity what we really mean. Certainly, except for actors or politicians, the movements we make with our shoulders, arms, and hands are spontaneous and largely unconscious. If you're curious about that, try consciously moving your arms while you speak. It feels simultaneously ridiculous and artificial.

But tomorrow, dawn will come...
She will look in at me with her thin arms extended,
offering a handful of birdsong and a small cup of light.

— William Collins

We see in sign language an entirely linguistic use. Similarly, in activities such as typing, musically performing, or painting, we are dealing in the realm of special languages and gesture.

Through touch, massage itself meaningfully bridges the manifestation of these two aspects—dynamic action and self-expression. We touch people with heartfelt care. We also give them nonverbal information, messages, and suggestions through touch.

On any given day, I may consciously convey various messages to clients. With someone who I sense is lonely, I may help them feel with a touch they are not alone. With a very firm touch, I may suggest to the person to feel how strong they are. For a person who considers their appearance unattractive, an honoring touch can connect them to their real beauty.

With touch, the person locked into his head can be made aware of the teeming and wondrous world of his body.

With a simple stretch, we can show the person with shoulder tension how tight they are, and by deepening the stretch, how much more freedom they can quickly enjoy.

Freeing the shoulder girdle is essential for the health of the hands, arms, and torso. As a therapist I often see people whose shoulder blades have become adhered to the ribcage. In structural and energetic theory we can see the ability of the shoulder blades to glide freely over the ribs as the literal and figurative basis for the freedom of the arms.

Without the open subscapular space, everyday stresses can become "impacted," instead of "rolling" off our backs, thereby affecting the excursion of the ribs, the free movement of the backbone, and ultimately the realm of the lungs and heart itself. As noted in the last chapter, at the level of the shoulder girdle, the vertical energy flowing through the body intersects with the horizontal flow through the arms and the hands, reaching out to the world around us. This may be seen as an axis of love.

A thinker collects and links up proofs. A mystic does the opposite. He lays his head on a person's chest and sinks into the answer.

— Rumi

Pectoralis Major

Enhancing wingspan is essential to the healthy life of the upper body. Thus the most important starting place is the pectoralis major.

If we think of the lower body as the root of our body-tree and the torso as the trunk, the shoulder girdles and arms are the branches. We need freedom in our branches.

Contact your sense of the majestic role that the shoulders and arms play in our lives. Center yourself and feel healthy in your own body, especially your upper pole and limbs.

Position yourself standing alongside the table, facing the client's upper ribcage.

Starting on the right side, use your right loose fist. Take it (fingers facing toward you) and place it on the sternum without pressure. You should be at the level of the upper ribs, usually ribs 1-4, well above the level of the breasts. Add a slight posterior pressure (toward the table surface) on the sternum and sternal ends of the upper costal cartilages, taking out the looseness. You don't need to press hard when largely on bone.

Without sliding over the skin, initiate a pull laterally, giving the nervous system an indication of the direction in which you will go. Add movement and direction laterally. Go slow enough, lengthening the pectoralis major with a deep effleurage, so that the client has enough time and breath to let go from inside out as you move. When you reach the area between the torso and the arm, clearly disengage.

Now place both fists alongside each other as if they were one wide fist, as medial as you can get on the humerus. You will likely be starting medial to the anterior deltoid.

Take out the looseness with a little posterior-ward pressure. Take up the slack, pressing deeper and initiating a lateral pull, without yet moving through the tissue. Now add additional vectors, by deeply drawing your fists laterally through the deltoid and deeper to the pectoralis major.

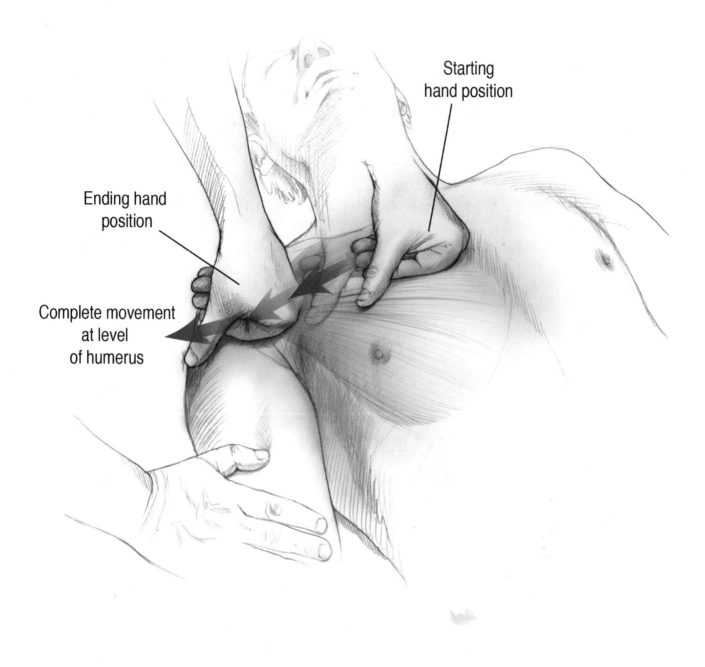

Starting
hand position

Ending hand
position

Complete movement
at level
of humerus

Figure **18**. Pectoralis Major − 1

The Deep Massage Book

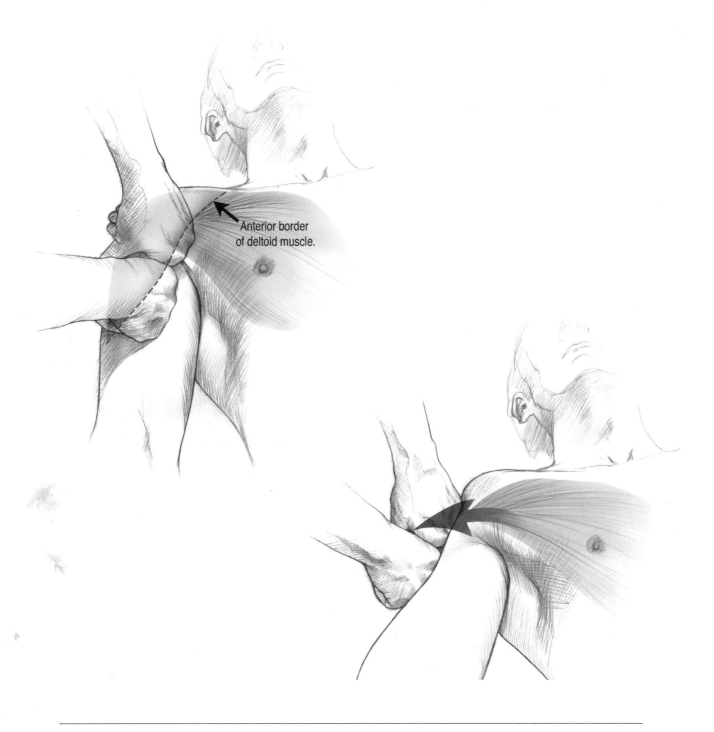

Anterior border
of deltoid muscle.

Figure 19. Pectoralis Major – 2

You will likely see the whole humerus rotate outward. That outward rotation of the arms reminds me of the "snow angels" children make, waving their extended arms while lying in fresh snow.

Maintain your effleurage as far out as you can. Often I will end up with my fists resting on the table surface. Do make sure you don't pinch the soft tissues as you move through the middle and some of the posterior fibers of these muscles.

Then move to the left side and initiate this fulcrum for the left side of the chest.

Biceps Brachii

The biceps play an essential role when we draw things toward us. Since they flex the elbow, every time we bring food to our mouths, every time we hug a friend or cradle an infant, the biceps are performing a life-nurturing service.

Think of what you would miss if you had the misfortune to have an arm amputated! Many people suffer from a lack of self-awareness and self-appreciation, and have very little consciousness or appreciation of their arms. Enjoy bringing an amplified awareness of life into your arms and to those of your clients.

As with all fulcrums, start by centering yourself. Stand alongside the right arm. Take the wrist with your right hand and lift it up so that the elbow is flexed at about 90°.

Place your left loose fist at the beginning of the upper arm, just beneath the shoulder. Gently at first, take out the looseness, pressing down toward the table. Gently take up the slack, tractioning the fascia without moving. Now add additional vectors, moving your fist down through the biceps. Do not go too deep here; a lot of pressure on the biceps, especially near the shoulder, can be irritating. As you get closer to the elbow, let the arm straighten a bit and continue the stroke across the elbow down along the radius, the thumb-side forearm bone, and end this fulcrum about two inches distal to the elbow.

Set the arm down in its extended length, clearly disengaging.

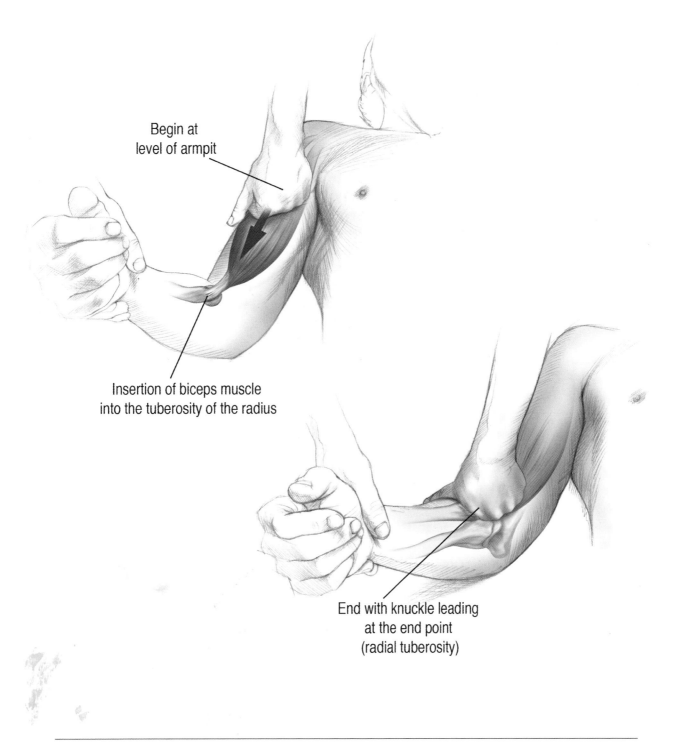

Begin at
level of armpit

Insertion of biceps muscle
into the tuberosity of the radius

End with knuckle leading
at the end point
(radial tuberosity)

Figure 20. Biceps Brachii

Triceps Brachii

The triceps straighten the arms, extending the elbows. Thus, they are pivotal in reaching out or in pushing away. Largely through them run the meridians associated with the fire element in Chinese medicine.

Again, center yourself, and stand alongside the client's right arm. The client is supine, with an arm raised over and alongside the head, with the inside of the elbow supported on a pillow.

Place your loose fist just beneath the armpit near the origin of the triceps. Take out the looseness. Then take up the slack, creating the beginning of a stretch toward the elbow.

Begin to add additional vectors, with a slow, deep effleurage. Continue until you reach the triceps tendon just at the top of the olecranon process. Pause, clearly holding the traction here. Clearly disengage.

Let the client relax into this new length, this new experience. Then reposition the arm alongside the body.

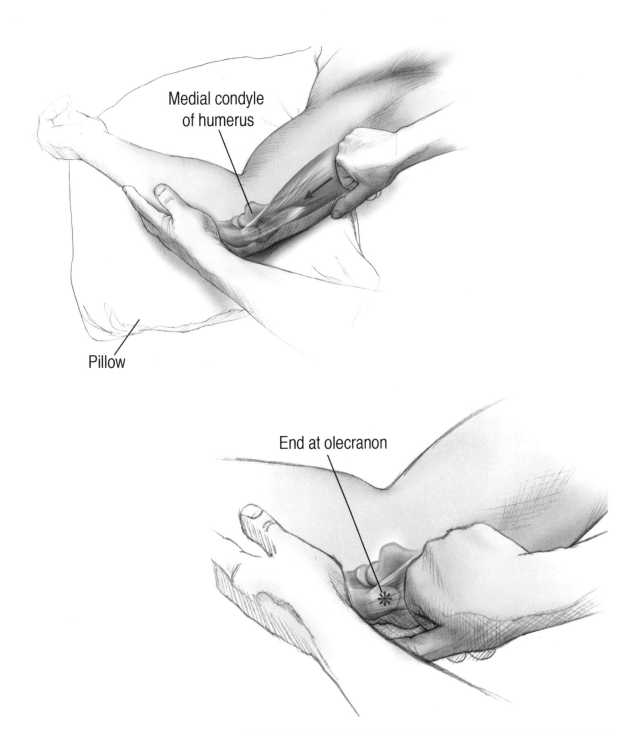

Medial condyle
of humerus

Pillow

End at olecranon

Figure 21. Triceps Brachii

Levator Scapula

The levator scapula, along with the trapezius, is a barometer for overall bodymind tension. One of the most common responses to stress is to elevate the shoulder girdle. I remember winters in Chicago. Sometimes my shoulders were up so high they could have been earmuffs!

Allowing the graceful descent of the scapula is fundamental to letting go of held-in stress. Know, when you are doing this fulcrum, that you are likely releasing stress that has been held for weeks or months, or possibly for many years.

The levator scapula originates from the side of the middle four cervical vertebrae C2-5. It inserts at the top of scapula medially, near the superior angle, the so-called "root" of the spine of the scapula. It is interesting to note that, to add strength, nature has this muscle twist as it ascends, a braided rope being stronger than just parallel strands.

The levator scapula is often chronically shortened, pulling up on its area of insertion. Muscles and fascia, even bone, will commonly thicken when there is a frequent pulling at a place of attachment. One of the body's most common fascial thickenings is the fibrous knot at the scapular attachment of the levator scapula. For most people, it is a sensitive trigger point.

Centering yourself, seat yourself at the head of the table and begin work on the client's right side. The client will be prone. Position your chair over the client's left shoulder. Face the right scapula. Place your right thumb near the superior angle of the scapula, with your fingers resting on the upper back. Wrap the fingers of your left hand around the lateral border of the scapula. Find the exact place of the usually thickened fibrous attachment of the levator scapula to the superior angle. Some people's scapulae are flexed forward so you sometimes need to go more anterior than you'd think to find the superior angle.

When you've found it (and often your client will say, "Yes, you've got it!"), pull the lateral margin up toward yourself while letting your thumb sink in gently, taking out the looseness.

One of the elegant aspects of this fulcrum is we get our pressure here not by pushing in hard with the thumb but by the lower hand pulling up on the lateral border, creating more looseness as the thumb simply sinks into the looseness thus created.

Pull up a bit more with the under hand (the left in this case) and take up the slack with the thumb sinking deeper into the insertion of the levator scapula. Make sure the area is not too tender—this should feel good!

Hold it... hold it... hold it... giving the client time in which to let go more and more deeply. Now clearly disengage.

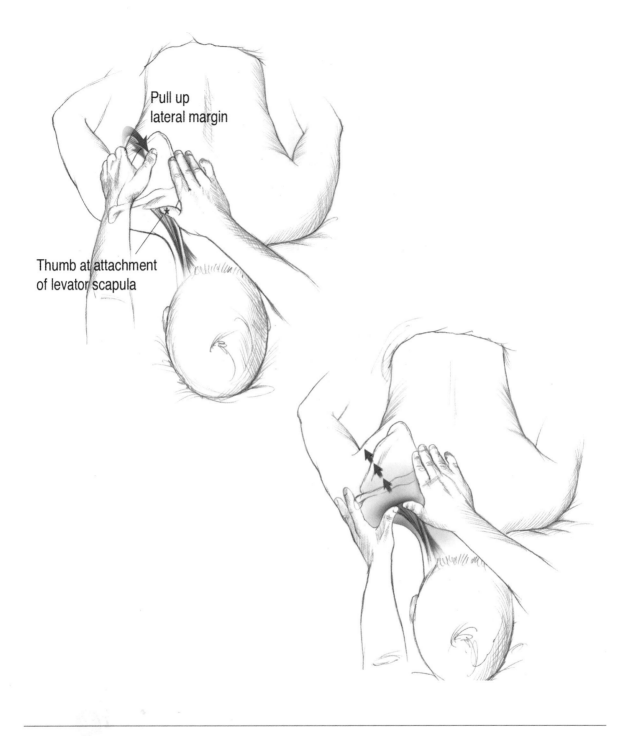

Pull up
lateral margin

Thumb at attachment
of levator scapula

Figure 22. Levator Scapula

The next step of this fulcrum is to give the levator a healthy stretch, a new experience of length, relaxation, and time; to let the nervous system come to a new "set point" with respect to this muscle's length.

Let go of the lateral border of the scapula. Take your left thumb and place it alongside the right thumb at the superior angle and medial upper scapula. The thumb pads should be placed facing inferiorly, so their contact on the top of the scapula is experienced as broad and fairly gentle. Let your fingers rest on the back, pointing generally in the direction of the right elbow.

Now take out the looseness, clearly contacting the attachment. Take up the slack, pressing into the attachment. Then add additional vectors, with the thumbs pressing the scapula down toward the elbow and taking it as far down as it can comfortably go without distorting the alignment of the client's torso. Rather than pushing with your thumbs and tensing the shoulder girdle, you can accomplish this movement just by letting the weight of your torso lean in.

Hold it… hold it… hold it. Give the client time to assimilate the experience of how good a fully descended shoulder girdle really feels; then clearly disengage.

Trapezius

For most people, the trapezius functions as the energy body's shock absorber, just as the feet and legs are the physical body's shock absorbers. Each time mild stress is experienced, the tension in the trapezius increases then quickly dissipates. Think of a resting cat when startled by a sudden noise. Its shoulders and other muscles instantly tense. The moment passes and the cat again relaxes and resumes its nap.

In situations where you have prolonged stress or experience a sudden overwhelming trauma, the body may absorb the stress, holding it instead of dissipating it. Then the trapezius (along with other common stress indicator muscles such as those around the eyes, jaw, and pelvis) may begin to have a chronically higher tonus. This diminishes our capacity to let everyday stress simply "wash off our backs."

Virtually every adult carries some tension in the trapezius with a resultant diminished capacity for absorbing everyday stresses. As a result stress becomes chronically lodged in this muscle. When our shock absorbers start losing resilience, stresses begin to hang on and potentially burrow deeper into the bodymind. In turn this can affect our breathing, heart rate, digestion, and overall muscle tone.

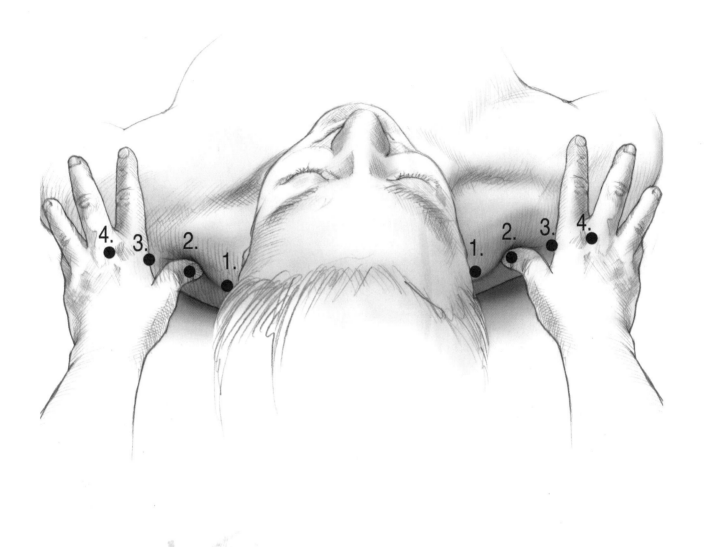

Figure 23. Trapezius Fulcrums

It is easy to experience stress in our busy lives. Merely in reading a newspaper, I can feel my trapezius tensing up. Often the pace of modern life is not well matched to natural biological rhythms. Our upbringings and societal expectations leave us with dysfunctional holding patterns that make us less able to cope with stress. I once read that we are all perfectly adapted to circumstances that no longer exist. We can overreact to things that should barely affect us simply because of past stresses that we haven't dealt with fully.

A primary purpose of working with the trapezius is to enable the letting go of any residual trappings that no longer serve us. We also want to encourage the new habit of handling stress by discarding it, rather than by absorbing it.

The form and name of the trapezius gives us information we need to do this. The trapezius comes from the same root as "trapeze." It refers to a four-sided figure. The trapezius originates along the body's centerline, as low as the 12th thoracic vertebrae and from each spinous process all the way up to the back of the head. It extends out finally to insert on the spine of the scapula and the lateral third of the clavicle.

The thickest part of the trapezius is its "belly" just above the scapula. It is from here that therapists can primarily sense how effectively shock is being absorbed or dissipated.

The healthy trapezius is like a sail that is optimally responsive to the winds of life. It allows the full excursion of breath underneath it, and for the freedom and healthy movement of the head, neck, and shoulder blades. Notably, a compromised trapezius will be thicker than normal—hypertrophied, especially in its belly. It will feel more like a hooded cowl, and be more yoke-like than winged. Let us restore our free-floating wings!

Center yourself before putting your hands on the client. Breathe. Position your body so that even when seated, you can use your body's weight and gravity, rather than effort, to attain appropriate pressure.

Position your treatment chair or stool to allow room between your body and that of the client. Let your joints be gently rounded, wrists aligned, elbows slightly bent, and shoulders and breath relaxed, with an open space between the outside of the rib cage and the insides of your arms.

Get grounded with ease in the hips and knees and the soles of your feet on the floor. If the client's neck is lordotic—chin higher than the forehead—put a small pillow under the head before you begin.

Briefly review in your mind the life stresses this client may have revealed in the pre-session interview/history intake and in past sessions if this is a repeat client. Realize you are not just touching the trapezius, a muscle positioned in the space of the client's body. You are equally touching time—

the accumulations of stress over a span of life. In this sense, every touch that impacts the client's ongoing life takes place at the intersection of space and time.

With the fulcrum model we are engaging the nervous system, especially the autonomic, as well as the physical structure.

Let your fingers rest on the clavicles and upper ribs. With your thumbs begin an exploration of the belly of the trapezius. Start near the base of the neck and work your way out with a mindful, caring touch, using light to moderate pressure. Note any associations and observations that palpating the client here evokes for you. Sometimes I feel like I'm a prospector, divining for long-lost treasures hiding beneath the surface tension. Work your way out in successive points near to where the clavicles and scapulae meet.

Now return to the belly of the trapezius, immediately lateral to T1. Be conscious of touching clearly with both your physical structure and your energy. Be mentally, emotionally, and spiritually attuned. Press in slowly with both thumbs, and then pause. You are now engaging the touch receptors.

If you find no tension, clearly disengage and explore points more lateral, but do make sure you devote some caring time and attention to each place.

If you do find tension on either or both sides, engage it with a bit more pressure. Commonly the client may say something like, "Now you've got it!" or you may see from their breathing and facial expression that they are engaged. Pause.

You are now engaging both the touch and pressure receptors.

Having entered their realm of tension, rest into it. First, rest yourself. Deepen your breathing. Sink in with your thumbs, lean gracefully in toward the client, letting gravity be the therapist, rather than forcing your way in by adding tension to your shoulder girdle, back, arms, or hands. Find the optimum depth for this fulcrum, this person, this place. Pause, without letting go of any vectors. Give the client some time in which to let go from inside out.

During this time it is important that you the therapist go to a "witness" state, not moving, patiently allowing the client to let go of successively deeper sedimentary layers of tension developed here over the span of his/her life.

At this point you are engaging receptors for touch, pressure, and the proprioceptors. Through them you are affecting the limbic system and possibly the cerebrum as well.

When you sense it's been long enough (five seconds is usually more than enough in a given place) clearly disengage and move on. Press in an inch more laterally on both sides. Repeat the steps above. Keep alive your sensitivity and patience. Clients need the gift of time and touch to let go of layers and years of accumulated tensions.

Continue working the belly of the trapezius in successively more lateral areas until you've given attention to at least four or five areas bilaterally. Even if you find more tension on one side than the other, maintain conscious contact with both sides. The bilaterality of contact is important since we are looking to restore the experience of having wings, rather than a yoke. Two wings are needed for flight!

Wonderfully, this fulcrum with the trapezius is physically quite easy to perform. Approached with reverence, respect, and patience, it will have global consequences for your clients. Through this nexus of time and space we are given the opportunity to let go of lifetimes of stress and to regain the sense of lightness in our lives.

The Mind in Bodywork: Understanding— The Sixth Dimension of Touch

We've explored the first five dimensions of touch—contact, movement, breath, graceful verticality, and heart. The sixth dimension essentially involves mind. Often we hear of bodymind therapy. But in what sense is what we do mindwork as well as bodywork?

I have never met a "bodyworker" who works solely on the body. Every single therapist I have met is, at least originally, inspired and thrilled to touch someone in a profound manner, in contact with the person, not just their tissues. Yet we don't often hear anything precise about the role of mind in bodywork.

Nick Lowe, an English musician popular in the 70s, aptly expressed the search for profound significance in his song, *"What's so funny about peace, love, and understanding?"* Whereas love comes from the heart, and peace from a grace that seems to vertically

descend upon us, understanding is properly the province of mind.

We ask, what is the role of understanding in bodywork? How may we come to truly understand ourselves and someone else? These are important and moving question. Their poignancy comes from the fact that there are limits to our understanding. We can never totally understand ourselves or anyone else.

Think how often your life seems an unfathomable mystery to you. Think about walking down the street and looking into a stranger's eyes and experiencing a sense of the nearly total mystery they are to you. Though I have been a teacher and a therapist for over thirty years, often I am aware of how little I feel I know. I think most teachers are relieved, surprised, and humbled that, in spite of all that we don't know, students and their clients benefit greatly from our work. I take this partly to indicate that, despite imperfect understanding, with just the first five dimensions of touch we can have a wonderfully positive impact.

Understanding necessarily requires a letting go of pretention. The limits and the gift of knowing include the grace of knowing how much we *do not* know. Just as life is bounded by death, like an island in the ocean, or a person walking down a quiet street, so understanding is surrounded by the vast unknown.

There is no need to despair at the limits of understanding. Remember that the very ability to consciously think, strategize, and choose is a truly miraculous empowerment.

To paraphrase Moshe Feldenkrais, who was a master of neurological bodywork, the uniqueness of the human nervous system is enough to qualify it as a new living function. The courageous effort to try to understand, to seek out the truth, is both an opportunity and a commitment for the dedicated therapist.

How is it then that we understand with our mind? It is through time, and through experience. Of the seven dimensions of touch, that of working with understanding is the first in which *time* is truly of the essence. As you work with your clients, as you cultivate your humility, patience, and courage, you will note how your understanding develops over time.

Taking a History

Understanding, of course, requires that we take a history. Notice the unusual choice of words. We may give a massage, but we take — we receive — a history. How can we explain this?

One of the greatest gifts we can give is our attention. In some respects, since our conscious, attentive nervous system is essentially a new living function, what we have uniquely to give is our attention. When we truly attend, when we fully receive a history, we commit to truly understanding someone else.

This understanding is not just cerebral. By itself, analytical attention is merely clinical. It maintains the illusion of objectivity. Although we do require whatever relevant analytical knowledge we can assemble concerning body, mind, and spirit, what we find is that true understanding always involves more than the conscious mind. When we truly understand someone else, we acknowledge input from gut impressions, subtle associations, intuitive hunches, and bodily felt senses of what it is like to be them. To really take a history we open into a space much larger than ourselves.

"Understanding" with our "mind" means an open awareness with the whole self, what the Zen tradition calls "Big Mind."

Taking a history means clearly receiving the impressions of someone else with one's mind, body, and spirit. If I feel their sadness with my heart I give it careful thought. I notice my spirit ascend as they reveal their hopes. I consider the clues offered by their past injuries, diet, medicines, books read, travels and exercises. Which therapeutic combination might help release their hidden potentialities?

Drawing on sensations, emotions, and thoughts, the therapist continuously composes whom they need to be to truly receive someone else.

Sometimes people forget that psychotherapy was originally called "the listening cure." Freud sat in a chair, out of view of the supine client, and said virtually nothing while the client freely associated. This curative power of listening is what we evoke when we open our whole selves to receiving someone's history.

Love means you breathe in two countries.
And skin remembers — silk, spiny grass,
deep in the pocket that is skin's secret own.
Even now, when skin is not alone, it remembers
being alone and thanks something larger
that there are travelers, that people go places
larger than themselves.

— Naomi Shihab Nye

The Massage of Time

Just as your body can palpate space and is designed to sense its interaction with space, so your mind is a sense organ designed to sense time. Without mind, there is no perception of time. When we receive a history and use it in the continuous process of illuminating our work, we are receiving time.

Time is the greatest gift. "I need time," we say. Perhaps we have enough time, though too often it may be devoid of spirit.

When we receive the history of a client, we can palpate not just the tense spaces in the body. We actually palpate *time* in the body, for time flows through us constantly as a nourishing river of "in-fluences," "in-flowings," from everywhere. We can detect the evolutionary struggles, failures, and achievements embodied in our genes, the unavoidable influences of our culture, the constricting and freeing influences of our family history, and not least, we can perceive the effect of decisions we have made consciously and unconsciously in response to these influences.

When we touch someone, we are touching these past tense times, the unresolved crises we physically enfold, the unresolved time of now. ***And we free them up!***—into the temporal energy flow. Our touch helps free the person to receive more deeply their own richness, the vast realms of possibility that course through their being.

Bodywork such as Rolfing (Structural Integration) helps integrate the body's structure. The alignment of each of our major segments, our spaces, is the great benefit of myofascial work. We can equally imagine that bodywork with deep understanding creates a healthier alignment of the *times* within the person's life. Massaging the person's "lifetime" as well as "lifespace" helps liberate no longer needed residues of difficult experiences and greatly amplifies healthy confluences from our past.

Time thus freed helps free the dreams of our ancestors—for in our cells and in our dreams dwell the unresolved struggles of humankind. "Temporal Integration" is a gift of massage with deep understanding.

The "Gospel" Form of Massage

Beyond taking a history and touching the client's space and time, how do we reach understanding? In the session, precisely how does understanding come about?

When I touch someone, I sense with my whole self their response: the nods, the groans, the frozen eyes of those steadfastly unrelaxed, the melting away of years in the facial expression. As therapists we encounter great variety in clients' affects and responses. There are talkers, complainers, snorers, oaken rigid people, the genial well. There are the unique grimaces, the bowel rumblings, the actions at a distance reported or sensed

by you, the deep relief of a breath-taking moment, the tears of internal thaw or joyful smiles, the arrival of serenity. An infinite litany informs us.

But what is usually taught to therapists? Only the motor skills to perform soft tissue manipulative techniques.

Our frontier explores the other half of the therapeutic realm—not that of our techniques but that of ***their world***, the vast world of the client's response.

As surely as we "call" with our skilled touch, the client "calls" back and responds at every moment in a completely unique way. Massage is like a chant, its essential form being call-and-response. Understanding arises out of this mostly nonverbal exchange, newly born from the dialogue of bodies and souls.

The actual practice of therapy has much more to do with the graceful, rhythmic back-and-forth swing of call-and-response than it does the unidirectional approach of diagnosis and treatment. People have studied the videographic archives of Milton Trager and Moshe Feldenkrais to determine what they did that made them such great therapists. Their observed techniques differed little from those of their students. However, one enormous difference *was* evident. They were observed to "track" the client moment-to-moment in a much deeper and more thorough manner.

The difference was in the listening. *For the call issues not primarily from us, but from the deepest dreams and hopes of the client.* When we truly listen and respond with understanding, it is more likely their dreams will come true.

The Harmonious Timing of Bodywork

We now know more about *how* we understand—through a history intake; through consciously touching time as well as space; through a call-and-response that builds healing interaction. But we need to know how to literally touch with understanding, and how a client might literally feel that understanding.

How does a client feel when touched empathetically by mind, not just by a hand? To feel truly healthy, to be truly at ease, people need to experience life with inner clarity, with the sense of understanding life more deeply than just with words. This comes about through therapy in which there is literally a meeting of minds.

Ida Rolf spoke of bodies as being too randomly organized. Such a remark is even more descriptive of the mind. Like bodily function, the healthy organization and life-enhancing function of the mind is essential to good health. The confusion that seems more and more epidemic in our world is something we can help dispel through healthy, thoughtful touch.

We are used to conveying understanding through words. In bodywork, since touch is our primary medium, we mostly don't use words. How can touch itself convey understanding without words?

When we touch, we are moving within the client's structural body and energy field. As we understand the client better and better, our movements become more and more appropriate responses to what we sense.

A session is going well when I almost effortlessly sense the invitation to move in—

when the client's breathing tells me to work in unison with them and for how long to take my hands off to give them a moment alone to savor or process their experience. The passive client may call for a stimulating tempo distinctly not in time with their lethargy. I intuitively give them a different experience: we share in refreshing and temporarily chaotic moments that present new possibilities for the nervous system.

Often the sessions with greatest understanding come when we work in entrainment—when both individuals share a sense of underlying timing, and attune more precisely to one another.

Indeed as humans we share rhythms of heart, breath, movement, and thought—we have much in common. Despite some allopathic pretense regarding logical treatment protocols, all forms of bodywork are still essentially improvisational. When two musicians improvise, the underlying rhythm is respected, while both are free to depart from it as far as they care to go, as long as the sense of coherence is retained.

In our therapeutic sessions we sense, through call-and-response, when we are on track, and when both participants are free to be who they are. Working together, we are also playing together. Health arises from this nexus of play and work. With this bodily felt sense of harmonious rhythm, dis-ease is replaced by a sense of ease and a clear knowing of self. Self-knowing is what is evident when we release the existentially chaotic rhythms of confused thought and feeling.

Understanding is expressed and created in bodywork by rhythmic movement. Meaning arises from rhythmically significant meeting. To quote Duke Ellington, "It don't mean a thing if it ain't got that swing."

In harmonious therapeutic moments, it is not merely our body that is swinging. Our mind is gracefully swinging as well. As we touch, we can notice our awareness fluctuating rhythmically from our own awareness of our body... to a key fact we remember from the client's history... to a relevant emotion we feel... to our palpatory sensing... to a remembered favorite technique for the supraspinatus... to a prayer we make to help us all get well.

The infinite swings of mind inform each body movement. So too the mind and the being of the client swing in turn gracefully through myriad places and times. By freeing the client in this way, we greatly expand not just physical range of motion, but also the range and movement of the soul.

As therapists, working with our minds, hearts, bodies, and spirits, we experience this swinging every single day. In mindwork as well as bodywork, the consciously evolving cosmos, in which we are a wild swinging element, is growing.

Between the poles of the conscious and unconscious,
there has the mind made a swing:
Thereon hang all beings and all worlds,
and that swing never ceases its sway.
Millions of beings are there:
the sun and the moon in their courses are there.

Millions of ages pass, and the swing goes on.
All swing! the sky and the earth and the air and
the water; and the Lord Himself taking form:
And the sight of this has made Kabîr a servant.

—Kabîr

Essential Connections

For most of human history, medicine has had an essential connection with spirituality. Until the 20th century, virtually all hospitals in the world were affiliated with a church, temple, or religious order. During this century, medicine and spirituality have stood somewhat farther apart. Though many medical practitioners are attracted to the "care" in healthcare, unfortunately the technological emphasis of 21st century medicine tends to separate "health" from "care."

Let us hope that the separation of spirituality and medicine is a temporary aberration. May we look back in twenty years and wonder how we could have ever lost sight of truth, just as we now shake our heads in amazement at how many doctors, until recently, heartily endorsed baby formulas and rashly dismissed breastfeeding. The profit motive—the manufacture and marketing of pills and machines—still dominates medicine. The unpatentable nature of the human spirit renders it of little interest to pharmaceutical manufacturers or insurance companies. Yet even in the massage therapy profession we have seen a tendency to tout the medical powers of our work while paying less attention to the spiritual.

Let us not forget that massage contributes something essential beyond its medical efficacy; it also embodies the spiritual component of human contact in healthcare. This is the strongest evolutionary leverage we have. When we touch, we connect, allowing the human spirit to soar, to rediscover the sanity of loving kindness toward ourselves and toward one another, and to take our evolution and our healthcare back into our own hands. In this way we can reclaim the realm of medicine from the insurance companies and drug manufacturers. We can match the technological progress of the last century with equal spiritual progress in this century, clearing a pathway to a much greater partnership based on a fuller understanding of the human body, mind, and spirit.

In the Beginning

In Genesis it says that Adam "knew" Eve. This is usually taken to mean "made love with." Let us rather consider that perhaps this divine and generative knowing is the same as the knowing in our work. When the therapist works with real understanding, the client senses that the therapist "knows" exactly what to do. *I am not just being well cared for, I am known. I am called by my true name.* When we are known in this sense, creation happens. When there is a true meeting of two spirits, minds, hearts, and bodies, the creation of a new reality occurs.

The theory of the "Big Bang" posits that creation happened a long time ago. It portrays the rest of the history of the cosmos as a kind of anti-climactic universal winding down. I prefer to perceive that creation is happening at every moment. At each instant the past disappears and the present is created afresh. There are new openings and always fresh possibilities for everyone. Every moment is an opening for creation.

The Biblical Genesis says, "In the beginning was the Word." This is depicted in Michelangelo's painting of God touching Adam and thereby imparting the spark of life. We may wonder, was God's creation through a word, an actual sound, or was it rather communicated through life-giving touch? Perhaps it is the hand of God that conveys the life-giving Word, inspiring each breathing being.

As massage therapists, our touch speaks to the client with our whole being. The promise of touch is to facilitate for everyone the creation of a new level of health. With our hands we give our word.

And in the beginning is the word.

Head and Neck—Anatomy, Energy, and Fulcrums

Loosen the knot of greed
so tight around your neck.
— Rumi

The neck is a key bodymind passageway. Nourishment passes down it through the esophagus to the stomach. Our breath flows in and out through the tracheal passage in the neck, giving us an even more fundamental form of nourishment. We can live without food for days, without air only a few minutes. Through the neck run the nerves connecting the brain to the limbs, torso, and visceral organs.

The neck is the meeting place of the heart and mind. One can see singing as being the audible convergence of heart and mind through the neck. In addition, the neck is the passageway for sound and speech. "Speaking from the heart" and "speaking one's mind" both rely on the neck. The words we

choose, the rhythm, the tempo, melody, and tone with which we say them, depend on the lungs, neck, and mouth.

The freedom and clarity of heart and mind in inward and outward expression are dependent on the neck, and are reflected in the individual's structural health. Imbalances here may commonly manifest as any of the following:

- Neck tension
- Neck compression—the eventual result of chronic muscle tension
- Exaggerated neck length—conveying the sense of mind and body only tenuously connected
- Head forward posture—straining the upper back muscles

- Posterior head (flat cervical curvature)—possibly from an overly rigid upbringing
- Vocal limitations—chronically soft or loud voice, exaggerated tone (e.g., whiny, shouting, teasing, husky, flat)

What does the head itself tell us? Sometimes too much! But certainly it is a most majestic and powerful center of being! I am in awe when I think of all that transpires in the head and the brain inside it.

It is certainly true that the head and its contents are highly valued in our society. Consider our distraction and preoccupation with our facial visage, or the inordinately mental focus of our education and our work. Yet in fact, body, emotion, and spirit have equal or greater influence on our lives—though they are often neglected compared to the focus accorded the brain.

Nonetheless, we do have here the realm of conscious thought, utilizing both the logical and imaginative sides of the two cerebral hemispheres. Deeper lies the limbic system, the diencephalon, the autonomic nervous system featuring the hypothalamus, the origin of the endocrine system, inhabited by most of our memories, deepest beliefs, hopes, dreams, and desires.

At the rear bottom of the brain we have the cerebellum, from where comes our ability for coordinated movement. Most of our brain and most of our body are organized around making useful movement.

As if the vast territories of the brain weren't enough, in this region we also have the cranium and face. Through the form and movement of eyes, brow, nose, cheeks, mouth, and jaw, the face gives us infinite information. Just the slightest tensing of our partner's jaw can coalesce all our attention. The face is the most expressive part of the person.

Kissing, talking, smiling, shouting, laughing, eating, drinking, yawning, sleeping, paying attention, being surprised, being afraid—every one of these fleeting or sustained behaviors shows us how the face may reveal our deepest of secrets. Just as the stars' light reaches us, enfolding the ancient and unknowable origins of the universe, so the face reveals the original and hidden nature of the individual. Through the facial features and the shifting constellations of expression, the whole history of the person can be intuited and contemplated by anyone educated and willing to become conscious of what we deeply know when we really *see* someone.

Our brain has developed the ability to read, largely through the face, the emotions of others. The eyes open unto the soul. If we commit to truly *seeing* someone, that in itself is healing. From earliest childhood onward, we naturally desire attention and affirmation. We want to be seen, to be known, and to be cherished by our loved ones and our caregivers.

If You Love the Body

If you love the body you must know the bone
that ribs and peoples it; deeper than flesh you feel
the beauty. That will last, simply as stone

upheaves in season where the winter rain
rakes asters and drooping cornstalks from a hill.
If you love the body you must know the bone

of fingers that touch, of the high case where the brain
lurks, of the deep knock and door and sill.
The beauty that will last, simply as stone

remains, is what you love when the blossom is gone —
petals and sepals and stem, roots and soil —
if you love the body you must know. The bone

smiles behind our faces when we frown,
knowing while the sweet flesh will not hold
the beauty, that will last, simply as stone

lasts, my love. For saying what I can
I ask forgiveness - in time we'll know it well.
If you love the body you must know the bone,
the beauty that will last simply as stone.

— Richard Tillinghast

Take the time to see your client's face and ask yourself what it is telling you.

Often you will see a face in which chronically held expressions have caused facial muscles and skin to assume a habitual tension, sometimes like a mask. Chronically held expressions ultimately affect even the shape of the underlying bones, the teeth, and the proliferation of neurotransmitters in the brain. As we let go of chronic tensions here, we go back in time, evoking the Zen koan, "What was your face before you were born?"

Often when observing a client at ease on the massage table as our session ends, I am struck by the restored sense of innocence in their visage. As the person disengages from their usual worldly strivings, they let go incrementally of the face, the masticatory muscles, the scalp, the brain and nervous system.

With Deep Massage of the face, their original face is finally revealed, fully at rest, reveling in turn at new landscapes through new eyes. Their Buddha nature shines through, clear and beautiful as a new day.

Structure

The spine rising up through the neck is surrounded by a number of muscle layers. Posteriorly, the major muscles are the trapezius, the cervical erectors (especially the semispinalis), the multifidi and rotatores, and between the upper cervicals and the head, the deep suboccipital muscles. Along the side and front, most palpable are the scalene muscles and the sternocleidomastoid.

Uniquely, the facial muscles do not insert into bone as do the other "skeletal" muscles. Facial muscles originate and insert into the connective tissues of one another. This accounts for their incredible plasticity and the infinite variations of expression that our faces manifest.

Underneath the facial muscles live the masticatory muscles, the masseter and temporalis. These can grip, rend, tear, and crush. They add deeper underlying power to the repertoire of facial expression.

Epicranius

We now come to the muscle that overlies the scalp, the epicranius. This muscle is divided most commonly into two or more parts. The back part is the occipitalis and the front part the frontalis. Occasionally one will also hear of the temporoparietalis, the part that goes from the top of the skull to the cartilage of the ears.

When looking at these parts, we see that the overall structure of this muscle is very much like the diaphragm. In the center is a flat tendon called, poetically, the galea aponeurotica, and from it fibers radiate in all directions—to the back of the skull, the eyebrows, and the ears.

Beneath the epicranius is the external connective tissue lying on the cranium. These layers of fascia in turn dive in through the sutures of the skull and become the internal fascia surrounding the brain itself and at this point are called the meninges. Here we may envision that we are not only working on the muscles and fascia but also on the bones, the fasciae beneath the bones, the meningeal tissue around the central nervous system, and the brain itself, deep to the cranial fasciae.

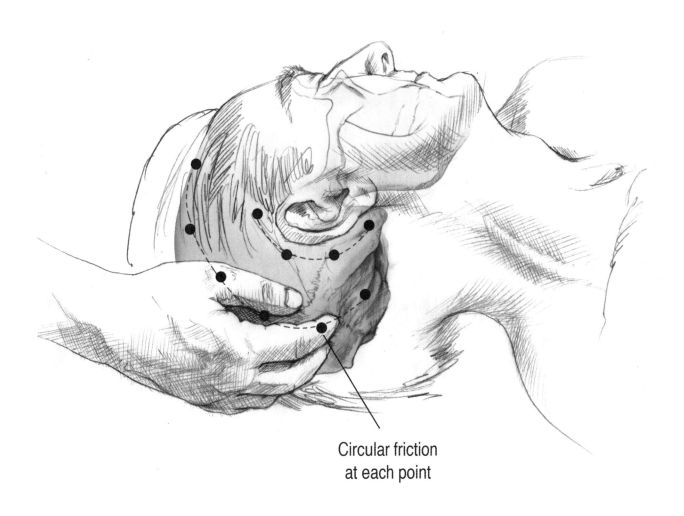

Circular friction
at each point

Figure 24. Epicranius

I believe the epicranius naturally reflects the history of the person's mind. The accumulated inspirations, efforts, and especially unresolved tensions can get lodged in this muscle that is closest of all to the brain. It is natural for the therapist to feel compassion for the tremendous and challenging work of each client's mind.

Center yourself. Stand at the head of the table. Cradle the head with your left hand, placing your thumb just above and a little in front of the ear and your palm and fingers resting on the skull behind the ear. Gently turn the client's head to the left. You may bend your wrist so that the client's forehead rests against the warmth of your forearm.

Place the fingers of your right hand behind the ear and at the base of the skull.

Take out the looseness, pressing in to the epicranius. Now take up the slack, pressing in a little more deeply, and visualize that you are in contact with the periosteum, the external fascia on the skull. Create additional vectors, making a half-moon semicircular movement with your fingers, tractioning the fascia.

Feel for the ease with which the tissues move. Feel for unusual changes of terrain—bumps, divots, ridges—that record the history of our cranium—all the stresses from birth onward: the falls off the jungle gym, the spills on the baseball field, last week's visit to the dentist.

Work each place relatively briefly. On the cranium anticipate the cumulative effect of a number of short fulcrums. The last thing you want to do is give a drilling sensation.

Completely disengage and re-engage a place about an inch to an inch and half higher. Repeat the steps above. Then choose another place just a bit higher and above the ear. Continue in a series of fulcrums ending above and just slightly in front of the ear at the beginning of the sideburn.

Now do similarly a second set of fulcrums starting at the base of the skull but immediately lateral to the centerline. This series goes from the back, to the top, to the front of the skull, to the beginning of the forehead just inside the hairline.

If we were to visualize in the landscape of Chinese medicine, we would say the first set of fulcrums is largely on the gallbladder channel and the second on the bladder channel that runs near the midline of the skull.

Set the head down and pause for a moment. With freshness and curiosity and care, repeat all the steps above working on the left side.

Consider what a blessing it is to relax the mind. Peace of mind more or less accompanies all our work. Paying close attention to the epicranius may especially deepen this peace, because of proximity to our center of thought.

The Face and Facial Muscles

The facial and masticatory muscles are designed to express emotion, to amplify sensation, to grasp, and to chew.

As noted above, the muscles of the face insert into the fascia of one another, not into bone. Elsewhere muscles through their tendons insert onto bone, attaching to the periosteal connective tissue covering the bone.

The muscles of the face are unique in the entire body: when one muscle contracts, it pulls on the fascia of one or more of the muscles around it. This gives origin to the vast range of facial expression that is more developed in higher primates than in all other animals.

The face is deeply expressive of our thoughts and feelings. Consciously or not, when we strive to keep our thoughts or feelings to ourselves, we naturally tense facial muscles or exhibit a lack of tone. Remarkably, not only is expression an effect of our thoughts and feelings, it is also a cause of them. Studies show that a grin, even when held artificially, will alter the brain chemistry to result in happier feelings.

The face also reacts to sensory input. Surprise or alarm causes us to open our eyes wide; distinctive scents flair the nostrils; a favorite food will evoke salivation. Apart from the sense of touch, all other sensory information is received through the face: seeing, hearing, tasting, smelling, even balance, which relies on the inner ear. The face is the aperture through which we perceive much of our world.

The muscles of mastication, while also expressive of feelings such as aggressiveness, have additional functions: to grasp, tear, and render what we eat unto the digestive system.

Massage of the face is not complicated. When we are fully aware of the profound roles the cranio-facial realm plays in our lives, we can bring deep respect to our quality of touch here—a touch that knows it is contacting our expressiveness, our thoughts, our emotions, our sensory world, our healthy aggression, and our nourishment.

In my practice and teaching, I prefer to use firm contact with the facial muscles. However, some therapists consider that stretching the facial muscles, especially with an older client, may further loosen the facial tissues. In this regard it is paramount to always respect the tastes and desires of your client, *doing only what they prefer.*

It is important to have freshly washed hands and forearms before you begin massaging the face. I recommend working without lubricant for better traction on the fascia, unless the client prefers otherwise. You may wish to consult with an esthetician for lubricant recommendations.

Center yourself. Begin by standing at the head of the table (to start); then sitting.

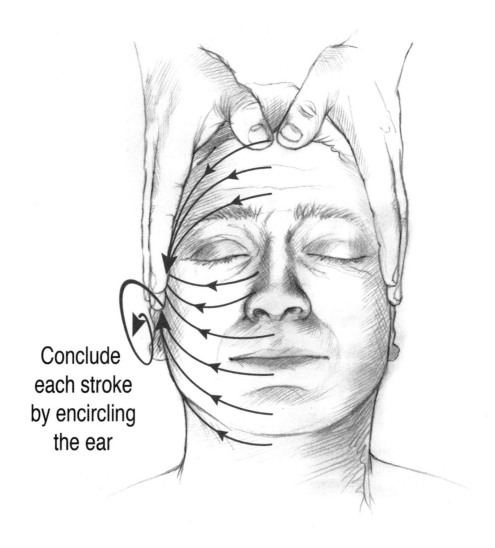

Conclude
each stroke
by encircling
the ear

Figure 25. Facial Muscles

The Deep Massage Book

Position the client supine with good support for the head (If you note more than the usual cervical lordosis, add a towel roll or small pillow to support the neck and head.)

Place your thumbs just below the hairline at the centerline. Take out the looseness, pressing down toward the table surface. Take up the slack, initiating a lateral traction between the thumbs without yet moving over the skin. Imagine, since the bone of the face is right up against the soft tissues here, that you are pressing somewhat gently into the periosteum, the connective tissue that covers the outer surface of the facial bones. Deep tensions may be detected here, lodged at the level of bone.

Add additional vectors, drawing your thumbs laterally away from each other, following just beneath the hairline. Ease up as you reach the temples and over the ears; then very gently go behind the ears and back up the face to the next point lower at the centerline.

Depending on the height of the client's forehead, complete three to five of these moving fulcrums, finishing with one that starts between the eyebrows and smoothes over the eyebrow area.

Now reposition to start just below the eyes. Generally you may find it easier here to work with the fingers rather than the thumbs. Continue with a series of fulcrums starting at the lower orbit of the eyes, outward from the base of the nose. Again go up above the ear each time to support the feeling of the face being uplifted. Then continue as above with fulcrums along the cheekbone, the upper jaw, the cheeks and the teeth lying deep to them, the lower cheek and the lower set of teeth, the side of the lower jaw bone, and finally a fulcrum on the undersurface of the jaw, the bottom of the mandible. With this latter pass, when you get to the most lateral aspect of the mandible, it usually feels best to go directly up behind the ear, through the place where the ear cartilage meets the cranium.

Each client is different. Some enjoy work on the ears, others distinctly dislike it. Please ask, rather than assume! Ask if they would like, for instance, four to five squeezes along the outer ear cartilage. If so, then feel free to squeeze or otherwise massage the ears. They are essential for listening and deserve to be included in our work—at the client's preference.

The Scalenes

The scalenes are embryologically the uppermost of the intercostal muscles—those muscles lying between the ribs that assist in inhalation and exhalation. However, there are no ribs in the neck! The scalenes actually originate from the "vestigial ribs" of the cervical vertebrae, and are visible as little buds on the cervical vertebrae. In fish, for instance, these would develop into ribs, but in humans they are merely small bumps to which the scalene muscles attach.

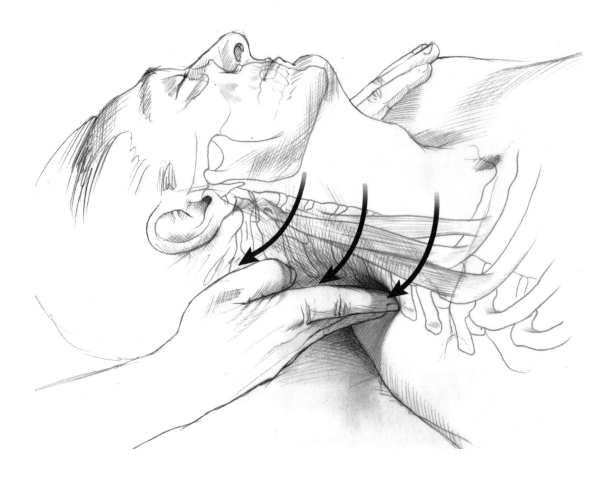

Figure 26. The Scalenes

Who would think about breathing with their neck? Yet scalenes have an important respiratory function. Some texts cite the scalenes as the second most important muscles of respiration after the diaphragm! They move the ribcage from above, while the thoracic diaphragm moves it from below.

The anterior scalene runs from the side of the second cervical vertebrae down to the first rib beneath the clavicle. Because it attaches to the front of that rib, the anterior scalene is one of the muscles that pulls the head forward. In addressing chronic head-forward posture it is important to include this muscle. The medial and posterior scalenes run more along the side of the neck and therefore have more to do with tilting the head to one side or the other.

It is common in whiplash that the scalenes are injured as the head is whipped forward then forcefully back. This sudden excessive stretch may slightly tear some of the scalene muscle and connective tissue fibers.

Energetically, the scalenes can be connected with all the virtues and challenges of the neck. The head forward posture can signify sadness, self-esteem issues, or reactions to recent or long-held defeats. General neck tension will also manifest in the scalenes. That tension points to the various reasons for inhibitions people can have about expressing themselves.

Center yourself. Seat yourself at the head of the table, and provide good support for the client's neck and head.

Working on the right side of the scalenes, place your middle finger, assisted by your other fingers, near the origin of the sterno-cleidomastoid, just above the sternal end of the clavicle. Press gently in and take out the looseness.

This fulcrum utilizes the active movement of the client: taking up the slack is begun by your client. Ask the client to lift their chin (without lifting their head off the table) just as if looking up. This will take up the slack, stretching the anterior scalenes in particular.

Add additional vectors, again in a movement partnership. Ask the client to slowly turn their head to their left, as if to look over the left shoulder. As they move, draw your fingers horizontally through the tissues on the right side of the neck. For this whole pass you are at the level of C6-7.

You may continue with your tractioning of the fascia all the way back as far as the spinous processes at the center of the posterior neck. In this case, you will have gone considerably past the scalenes, but you will be more completely addressing the soft tissues of the neck, pulling them back. As a result, the head will come back more on top of the body instead of projecting out in front of it.

Now ask your client to bring their head back to center. Begin a second fulcrum at the level of the middle of the neck, around C3-5. Repeat each of the steps above.

Finally, ask your client to return to center again, then begin a third moving fulcrum at the level of C1-2. Repeat the steps above. Then switch your working hands and address the scalenes and posterior neck similarly on the left side of the client's neck.

Posterior Neck

The back of the neck or the neck of the back? It was a toss-up whether to include this next series of fulcrums in the back section or the neck section of this book. However, as readers it would seem odd to study the posterior neck in the back chapter rather than here—even though nature basically doesn't know we think we have a neck.

The posterior neck muscles are for the most part back muscles. Indeed the spine extends from the tailbone up to the occiput. Some books even contend that the bones of the cranium are themselves simply irregularly formed vertebrae. The brain and spinal cord are continuous, just as the spine and head. A well-functioning neck is simply the upper aspect of a long, free, healthy spine.

Like the "Nine Points" in Chapter 7 (The Back), working with the posterior neck proceeds systematically through layers. Sometimes when working with the layers of tension in the body, I have the distinct impression that they are like the sedimentary layers of the Earth. The surface is of most recent origin, with deeper layers comprising past surfaces from some time ago, and the deepest layers, compressed under many others, representing even earlier times.

The deeper we go into the body's space, the farther back we go into its history.

Deeper in space equals deeper in time. As I've learned from Zero Balancing, we can logically assume that the deepest tensions may be held at the level of bone, our most dense living layer underlying the muscles.

In the posterior neck you have a number of layers. Let me mention the first three layers I find clinically most significant.

The first layer is the trapezius muscle. Recall this originates along all the spinous processes down to T12, as well as at the back of the occiput.

Deep to the trapezius the next most important layer is the cervical portion of the erector spinae muscles—the iliocostalis, the longissimus, and thickest in this region, the spinalis. The spinalis fuses here with a deeper muscle called the seminspinalis capitis. It is the thickest and strongest of the posterior neck muscles.

Deep to the erectors are the multifidus and rotatores. These originate on the transverse processes and travel obliquely up to the spinous processes, the multifidus originating also on the sacrum.

There are yet deeper anatomical layers and fulcrums in the posterior neck not described here. They require hands-on palpation and supervision and are thus best left to the classroom arena to assure clarity.

Posterior Neck 1. Trapezius (prone)

Initially sit or kneel alongside the client's head. The head will be tilted down a bit in an adjustable face cradle.

Place your thumb just along the lateral margin of the trapezius at the base of the neck, at the level of C7. Take out the looseness, pressing medial-ward and slightly deeper. Now add additional vectors, drawing your thumb through the trapezius slowly to the midline, to the spinous processes. Clearly disengage.

Then re-engage and, in the same manner as above, do this moving fulcrum through the trapezius a total of four to five times, each pass a bit higher than the last.

This series of trapezius fulcrums is not very deep. They set the stage for deeper work and help the head come back on top of the body. Because I view the trapezius almost like a curtain behind which transpires the more serious drama of the neck muscles proper, I call this series of fulcrums "Lifting the Curtain."

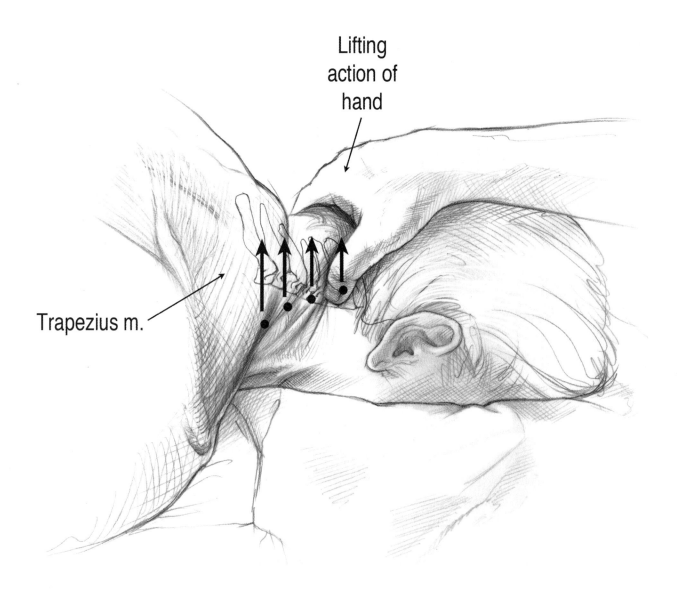

Lifting
action of
hand

Trapezius m.

Figure 27. Posterior Neck 1 — Trapezius

Posterior Neck 2 — Semispinalis Capitis

Start again at the base of the neck. Place your thumbs a little deeper and lateral to the trapezius, about one-and-a-half inches lateral to the midline and about a half-inch toward the front of the body. You will be pressing in toward the bodies of the spinous processes.

Press medially into the belly of the semispinalis capitis. Take out the looseness and first palpate for tension. Draw your thumbs from the front to the back (anterior to posterior) across the grain of the semispinalis fibers and feel for tension. If you find no tension, clearly disengage and move on to the next higher point.

If you find tension, take up the slack with a little bit of pressure medial-ward. The neck is considerably more delicate than the back, so please err on the side of gentleness when it comes to your pressure here.

Melting into the tension, add additional vectors by resting in just a little more deeply and holding while you relax and breathe, allowing the client time and space in which to relax and release from inside out. Then clearly disengage.

Repeat as above, with fulcrums as called for, in a total of about five areas here, each slightly higher than the last.

Posterior Neck 3 — Multifidus/Rotatores

Start again at the base of the neck. Place your thumb halfway between the tip of the transverse process of T1 and the spinous process of C7 (Figure 29). You'll be pressing into this "transverso-spinal" group of muscles, entering the neck muscles from a 45° angle.

Take out the looseness. Palpate for any tension by drawing your thumb up across the grain of these fibers. Since they run obliquely across the vertebrae, it is clearest to palpate from inferior to superior, as if you were drawing your thumb across the rungs of a ladder. If you find no tension,

clearly disengage and move on up to the next vertebral level.

If you do find tension, take up the slack with a little bit of pressure postero-medially. Melt into the tension, adding additional vectors, resting in just a little more deeply into the lamina groove and holding while you relax and breathe, allowing the client time and space in which to relax and release from inside out. Clearly disengage.

Repeat these steps as called for at each vertebral level until you have covered the area, with your last contact being between the C3 transverse and C2 spinous processes, where these muscles end.

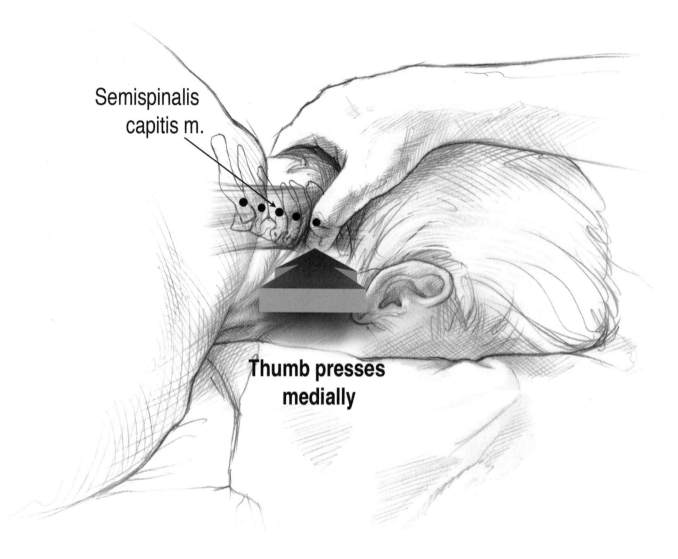

Semispinalis
capitis m.

**Thumb presses
medially**

Figure **28.** Posterior Neck **2** — Semispinalis Capitis

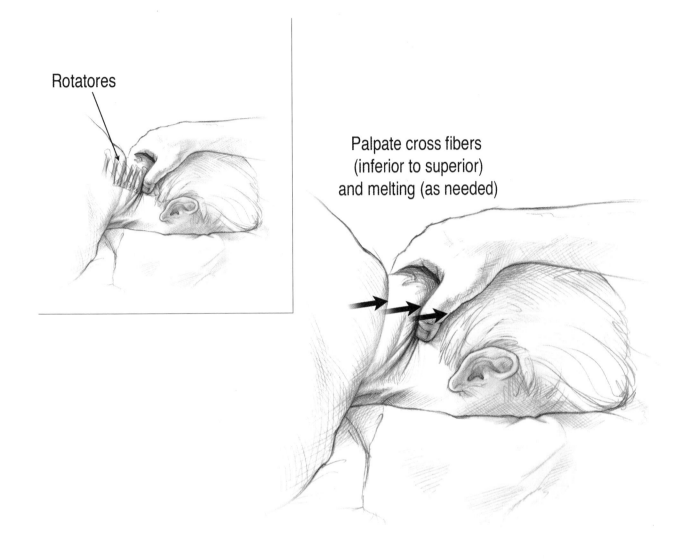

Rotatores

Palpate cross fibers
(inferior to superior)
and melting (as needed)

Figure 29. Posterior Neck 3 — Multifidus and Rotatores

Half-Moon Vector through the Neck

Like the Half-Moon Vector through the Legs, this Half-Moon Vector is explicitly a field fulcrum. It is not aimed at a specific place. Although we are clearly at interface with the occipital bone, the fulcrum is experienced by the client globally through the neck and often through the spine, torso, and quite frequently through the whole bodymind.

Letting go of our heads can be physically and psychologically challenging. Most of us behave as if thinking were the most important thing we did. Descartes, we recall, said, "I think, therefore I exist." Being, of course, has much greater scope than just thinking. For all the much-touted mind-body connection, it also can be healthy to experience some spaciousness in the mind and body relationship. When we traction gently on the occiput, a healing space opens up in which we can let go of the mind's loud pre-occupations and hear the quieter voice of the whole self.

There is a tributary of energy deep inside us, in our very bones. It is called various things by different traditions— *élan vital, kundalini, nadis, qi*, core bioenergy, universal life flow, central nervous system. Take your pick. When we experience that deep flow, we simultaneously feel sanity restored. Deep inside, we know we are all a part of the larger universe.

The isolated self is in some respects an illusion, as is bodily separation from the environment. We are interdependent. The life that we have is not our own creation, it is a flowing realization of genetic potential in time. Creation makes life again and again, producing this tree of life in which we live. For all its vaunted narrations, conscious mind is not in control. It is a tool and at that a tool too often inflated in its self-estimation, taking up more than its fair share of energy.

The writer Lewis Hyde said, "Our gifts rise from pools we cannot fathom." With Deep Massage we sink down into the pools from which our gifts arise. We refresh and balance our clients—and ourselves—anew. Life is more fully lived with each fulcrum into this field of energy that deeply constitutes and nourishes us.

Center yourself as you begin, seated at the head of the table. Place your hands under the client's head. With your fingertips find the undersurface of the occipital bone. The occiput has a posterior surface. At the bottom of that surface, it travels anteriorly, actually ending as far forward as the jaw! You are looking to place your fingertips just on the beginning of that underside. Make sure you are not pressing into C1 or C2; it is important that you're at interface here only with the occiput.

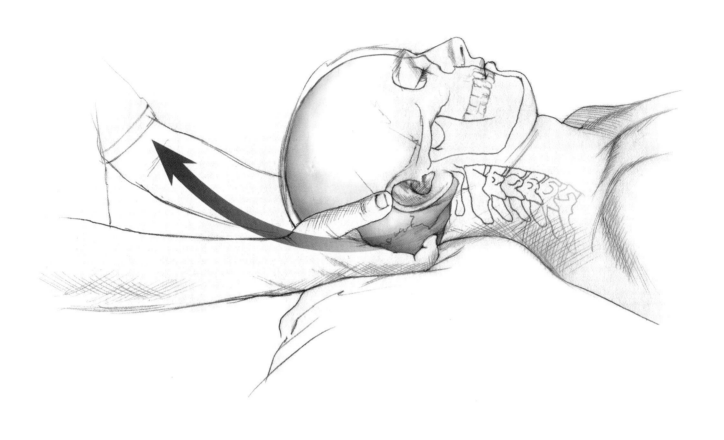

Figure **30.** Half—Moon Vector through the Neck

Let the back of the head naturally rest on your palms and fingers. Nestle. Spend some time with your fingertips gently locating a really clear bone-to-bone connection with the inferior border of the occiput and then gently taking out the looseness in the neck.

Now put in the Half-Moon Vector. Do this by simply bringing your fingers more toward yourself. This will add additional gentle traction and a slight flexion of the head on the neck (the chin should incline very slightly toward the chest).

Hold it... hold it... hold it. Allow the client to relax their mind, body, and spirit.

When you sense it's time to let go or when you see a working sign, set the head and neck down in length. It's important for the client to be left with an open, lengthened feeling.

Allow the client some moments to savor the experience, then move on in the session.

Just as with the Half-Moon Vector through the Legs, this is a fulcrum you can repeat a few times during upper body work. It is deeply centering and integrative of the other work you have done.

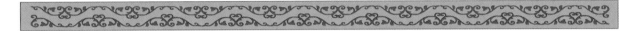

Part Three

Alchemy—
the Seventh Dimension of Touch

It is good science to work with what is real. For humans what is real is our three-dimensional bodies of length, breadth, and depth, within which we experience sensations, emotions, thoughts, and, however you choose to conceive of it, spirit. In bodywork we naturally touch all these things.

The dimensions of touch we explored in the previous chapters are:

- **Contact**
  Using touch we literally establish a point or area of contact, an honored meeting place of two conscious beings.

- **Movement**
  When we initiate thoughtful movements with our hands, the client and the therapist attentively engage in a healthy exploration of self—the "two-dimensional" curving paths that constitute us.

- **Breath**
  When the therapist breathes freely, a higher level of energy comes into play within the session. Through breathing more deeply, both therapist and client experience their three-dimensionality. Through the living example of the therapist, the client in turn senses permission to be more fully alive.

- **Graceful verticality**
  Western physics and most energy models see the body's work/energy flow as being organized in a vertical orientation. Standing and moving with graceful verticality raises the therapist's energy level. In turn, this is experienced by the client as a heightened energy flow through their own body. Good biomechanics is also good energy mechanics.

- **Heart**

  When the therapist truly cares for the client in a way that is clear and palpable, the client experiences trust, literally feeling cared for within their body. They experience more love within themselves.

- **Understanding**

  When the therapist makes the effort to truly understand the client, and attends carefully during the session, the client feels understood. This translates not only into an experience of deeper physical ease, but also a letting go of confusions that may trouble their soul.

The seventh dimension, which I call alchemy, is, ironically, the one that is most "out of our hands." By alchemy I am referring to a client's experience of psychospiritual and somatic transformation as a result of being touched, much as gold is produced from lead in alchemical lore. As therapists we are human alchemists. Your most treasured experiences as a therapist will likely involve assisting such transformations.

At such moments we may feel that we are merely midwives to a natural process. When our clients experience a metamorphosis, it is much like assisting a birth. Both therapist and client are filled with a sense of awe and humility at the new experience of being that our connection brings into the world.

The earlier descriptions of the six dimensions of touch outline a psychosomatic technology for achieving this qualitatively higher level of health—the real meaning of massage/bodywork. But the actual step, the movement of the self into a new world of health, is out of the conscious control of the therapist. It is a decision initiated by our clients from deep within themselves.

Therapists facilitate the alchemical role of touch, simply by attending to the previous six dimensions. Beyond this, as the philosopher Ludwig Wittgenstein said, we must be silent. We let go. Just like the midwife, we perform all the preparations; then we allow nature to accomplish what remains to be done. The art and the science of letting go is perhaps the highest definition of touch therapy.

Understanding and practicing the skill of letting go involves five essential steps:

1) recognize the limits of speed
2) slow down
3) stop
4) rest
5) choose a new path.

Let us first fully acknowledge the limits of speed.

The Epidemic of Hypersympathetonia

"Hypersympathetonia" (HST) is a word I coined to describe one of the primary conditions addressed by massage therapy. It refers to a tendency for the "set point" of the autonomic nervous system to be tuned overly much to the sympathetic— the fight-or-flight part of the nervous system. HST is the natural biological consequence of being a people almost totally uneducated in rest.

HST is a phenomenon determined by our history, our culture, and its interface with our biology. The Industrial Revolution unquestioningly valued the ever greater speed of production. The Information Revolution even more dramatically worships the speed with which information can be processed. In this broadly accepted culture of instantaneous information procurement, it is natural to believe that we just can't think, act, acquire, or feel fast enough.

At times it seems we are hopelessly competing with the pace of computers. Remember the ballad of John Henry, who "died with his hammer in his hands," while attempting to compete with a jackhammer. Is there to be a similar expiration of the human mind?

HST is also affected by one of the primary tenets of consumerism: only what you don't yet have is worth having. This easily translates into the culturally pervasive sentiment that only *who we are not yet* is worth being. This combined conviction— that we do not have and are not what we need—feeds a mode of desperation in many of us. We try to become who we think we should be, and to get what we don't have. All the while we are trying to match the tempo of our computer-modeled relationship to time.

There is a shortlist of the biological and social costs of such beliefs. In HST, circulation is shunted away from the internal organs, causing them to become relatively dehydrated and undernourished. As a result, digestive and assimilative problems of all kinds multiply. It is telling that the majority of pharmaceutical aids sold worldwide are for intestinal distress. With reduced fuel for assimilation, every single cell in the body becomes undernourished, setting the stage for a plethora of chronic diseases.

At the same time, the heart and blood vessels suffer from overstimulation, since with HST the body is continuously readying itself for fight or flight. This predisposes us toward heart and circulatory problems. The endocrine system becomes out of balance as well, awash in norepinephrine and other sympathetomimetic hormones that accompany chronic stress and affect every cell in the body. This in turn may trigger a variety of metabolic, immune, and reproductive disturbances.

HST is implicated in the prevalence of insomnia and the attendant physical and psychological problems. The musculoskeletal complaints that contribute to a majority of worker absenteeism correlate directly to the neuromuscular system's constant readiness for flight or fight.

The mental and emotional consequences of HST are vast, contributing to attention deficit disorder, recurrent bouts of anger and fear, and even substance addictions to fuel our frantic doing or to artificially propel us into the parasympathetic when we just can't take it any more.

HST clearly fits the dimensions of a social epidemic. It is a major factor in accidents, in diseases born from exhaustion, in mental problems, and in person-to-person violence. Imagine the total economic cost of HST! It may well define the single greatest individual and social health challenge we face.

The Evolution of Slowness

Deliberation is born of joy.

— *Rumi*

Recall that Andrew Taylor Still, osteopathy's founder, said that the body contains all the healing substances it needs. Indeed humans have the antidote to HST within their nervous systems. The autonomic system embodies the advantage of a speedy, whole body response to changing circumstance.

However, we have evolved a yet higher capacity. Even during the most trying of circumstances, we have the ability to sort through our feelings, our thoughts, and our sensations and to consciously determine our response. This ability to make deliberate decisions is perhaps our most uniquely human characteristic.

Between stimulus and response there is a vast expanse. This is the unique capacity of the human cerebrum.

With our conscious mind, we can slow down our processes and choose who we want to be and how we want to act, as opposed to speedy and automatic reactions that characterize all lower levels of the nervous system. The ability to consciously slow down is one of the great privileges of being human.

Massage therapists and bodyworkers are an advocacy group precisely trained to facilitate the social necessity of slowing down and contemplating our situation and our habitual responses, then making deliberate, balanced responses.

A whole hour spent not moving but not asleep is the sacred hour spent in a bodywork session. It is a whole hour filled with contemplation, a whole hour spent outside of the rush of the everyday. It introduces a unique and significant window of change for our quality of life. The joyful experience of being out of the normal experience of time and mind and body is an evolutionary lever of tremendous power.

For our clients we need to expand not merely their physical range of motion, but their psychic range of motion as well. Most people spend their time either in a rush of activity or fast asleep. What if we had opportunity to explore the fertile mid-ground between sleeping and waking?

Historical accounts tell us that Thomas Edison had the habit of resting with his arm extended and a rock in his hand. When he fell asleep, the rock would drop to the floor and wake him. Gradually he got to where he could be almost asleep but not drop the rock.

Why? It was out of this vast but rarely explored realm between asleep and awake that his inventive genius stirred! Between the strictures of the conscious mind and the dream-saturated realm of sleep, he cultivated the state in which the fertile meeting ground of conscious and unconscious could yield its fruits.

The ability to be unhurried and at peace with our decisions may well be precursors for the further evolution of humankind. Automatic, autonomic reactions only reintroduce existing problems and our dysfunctional, habitual responses to them.

Perhaps, in this new century and beyond, we will avoid the repetition of past shortcomings; and instead make spiritual and humanistic progress that will trump even our technological successes. For this, the capacity to slow down is paramount.

Stopping the World

With slow and deliberate motions of our hands, and well-timed pauses, we slow down the client's world to empower inner deliberation; we may even help stop the world altogether. In Carlos Castenada's books, his Yaqui tutor don Juan Matus spoke of the necessity of "stopping the world." From time to time we need not just to slow our world but to stop it all together and start completely afresh.

Every time we still our hands during a massage or disengage our touch we allow the client a time of absolute rest within the overall flow of the session. We facilitate the creation of a new world, for such relaxed, sustained resting places seem to last an eternity, and usher in magical "clearings," openings in the field of energy and structure within us.

It is the same with music, where moments of silence, long tones, and held notes allow us to glimpse a world of infinite possibility. The times of complete rest within a massage session are moments in which the infinite hope and possibility residing within the experience of sacred time flow into us.

Bodywork modalities that facilitate the contradictory experience of nothing actually happening hold enormous social and evolutionary power. In Zero Balancing, for example, a number of specific vectors of force are sustained with absolutely no movement. When the practitioner holds a movement, it is like eternity in the palm of your hand: the world stops. Cranial work in which the therapist doesn't move, but rather is moved by the client, evokes the Muddy Waters transcendent song of love: "She moves me, man, but I don't see how it's done."

The Reiki therapist is in some sense motionless, tranquilly allowing healing energy from within and without to accomplish what is necessary. These and every resting moment in any mindful bodywork therapy take advantage of the archetypal power of stillness, of stopping, to help us change— for to change what we are doing, we must stop what we are doing.

What stops us—right in our tracks— forms the basis for memorable new experience. That in turn forms the basis for taking a new track, embarking on exciting journeys on roads not yet traveled.

Divine Relaxation

In the Bible it says, "And by the seventh day God completed His work which he had done ... Then God blessed the seventh day and sanctified it, because in it He rested from all his work." How did he do it? (Being God, he must be fantastic at resting!) Perhaps the biggest clue regarding the Divine form of rest is the statement concluding each day of creation: "And God saw that it was good."

Such contemplative self-realization likely holds the key to the direction we must take to truly rest. When we notice that with our best efforts and the enhanced wellness of our clients, it is truly, beautifully, and ethically good, we come to a profound and necessary peacefulness in our work. After a session, we can see that it is good. We can completely forgive ourselves for imperfections while striving nonetheless to grow in every way we can.

Carl Jung said that if we do not celebrate our successes, we become sick. The obvious corollary is, if we celebrate our successes and truly see that "it is good," we—and our clients—become increasingly healthy.

In *Seven Habits of Highly Effective People*, Stephen Covey, a modern guru of organization, tells us everything is created twice. First, we make a plan; second, we take the actual steps to accomplish it. Note, after all, that really everything is created three times. There is the thought, then the accomplishment, and then, if it is truly to live in the world, the letting go of the accomplishment. Nothing can be truly given, be truly alive, unless it is released in love. Care-giving is

doing the best we can and then letting go of it completely. Then we truly rest. Then we share perhaps the greatest gift of all—the gift of peace.

How long might we suppose the days of Creation lasted? God, after all, is not on Eastern Standard Time or Central Standard Time. He's on GST—God's Standard Time! How long was the seventh day? Perhaps the seventh day is both bound and unbound by time, much like the ideal spirit with which we let go in our work.

God created and then he rested and made that day holy. Perhaps—and it does appear this way—the entirety of time has transpired within this seventh day. Thus the Holi-day, the Healing Day of rest, is the one in which all our time is lived. If God is everywhere at every time, what space, what time, what day, is not holy? Thus we can aspire to resting in every moment, since every moment lived transpires in this holy day.

The Bodily Experience of Divinity

Our clients say it again and again: on the table they sometimes feel contact not just from the therapist. They feel as if an angel were deeply touching into them. This is, I believe, a far more common experience than is given voice. The bodily felt experience of divine touch is a natural though not

consciously willable result of mindful bodywork. Divine touch is by definition life-giving and alchemical.

Into the peaceful places and times within us shining grace descends, lifting us to new heights. Within this special time and space we pass beyond the realms of understanding and of learning. Thomas Moore says that the soul doesn't learn, it transforms. The metamorphosis of soul that accompanies enlightened touch is nothing we can exactly learn how to accomplish. Our deepest gifts arise from pools we cannot fathom. But arise they do, and this alchemy, this giving peace a chance, is what gives our profession its greatest power.

Deliberation leads to joy and joy to liberation. This is not a gift we keep. It is the great gift that we may pass on through the whole of creation simply by letting go.

Session Design

Intelligence is nothing more than discussing things with others. Limitless wisdom comes from this.

— Hagakure: Book of the Samurai

Integrating

Deep Massage, like Rolfing, cranial work, Zero Balancing, and other integrative styles of bodywork is a stand-alone therapy that can easily constitute the entire content of a session or a series of sessions. I certainly recommend you practice many sessions of pure Deep Massage until you can do the protocol that is given later in this chapter.

Practice until it is second nature. Practice until your body, mind, and spirit are focused naturally on sensing your client, and no longer on remembering the next fulcrum and how it's done.

Please feel free to integrate other modalities with Deep Massage. For instance, some clients may have the expectation of lubricant and Swedish-type strokes. Meet them where they are, adding a minimal amount of lubricant and using effleurage, petrissage, or rocking, which work very well before and/or after the Deep Massage fulcrums to integrate the part you've worked on into the whole body experience.

Alternatively, we can sequence Deep Massage. For instance, commonly I will do Deep Massage prone, then a full Zero Balancing with the client supine.

You might consider Deep Massage followed by a brief craniosacral protocol. You might also incorporate stretches and other body mobilizations at each body segment. I have heard of a study that showed deep work accompanied by stretches had a longer lasting and more profound effect.

Of course, the point is to interface with the person, to actually meet them. It is the meeting that is healing, not the intention to heal. It is your delightful job to do whatever it takes to best meet this individual. Don't just habitually deliver your favorite modality, whatever that may be. When a person asks me what kind of therapy I do, I ask them to say their name. If it is "Bob," I say, "I do Bob-therapy."

Use session design to meet the person.

Individualizing Session Design

Even anatomically, every client we work with is fully unique. The muscle and bone and every inch of skin has its own individual form and history. If they could converse, the organs, tissues, bones, and skin would tell us a compelling and unique story.

When fully grasped and understood, every person's life holds the fascination of a great novel. I am intrigued and humbled by each client! How do I access and draw out their true self, how might I most helpfully allow it to be?

Designing individualized sessions is a high art and science—one of the most profound endeavors we can undertake. Assisted by thinking, feeling, observing, and talking, we attempt to determine what interactions through touch will make an optimum difference in someone's life.

Asking yourself what is called for can be a bit overwhelming. How can we touch so as to liberate the action potentials of that client's story? Some client's requirements seem rather transparent, others more complex or tangled. In all honesty, there are days when we ourselves may not be as insightful as on others.

One piece of extremely good news is this: although each person is different, each person is also similar! Though different in precise form, each person has the same muscles and bones, the same overall anatomical and physiological organization. This enables us to immediately clarify our focus. For instance, if we know we will be concentrating on the back in a certain session, images of the relevant muscles—the latissimus dorsi, trapezius, rhomboids, erector spinae, multifidus, quadratus lumborum—float into our awareness and give us an itinerary for the session's journey.

Each person is already a coherent symphony of being. When we hear their song, we can improvise a session that harmonizes the music of their life.

All relationships are improvised. We forget this, especially with friends and loved ones, because we develop habits of relating. Ultimately, however, a relationship is a moment-to-moment improvisation. What will I say next? How shall I look at this person? What might they say next? What arm gestures will accompany this conversation? We know none of this in advance as we embark on a conversation.

Certainly, in therapy as well, everything from the first conversation to the last session is improvised. This reminds us to remain optimally awake and alive through each stage of the therapeutic process. Session design is not something done before beginning work at the massage table. It is not making a plan and sticking to it. Session design is something we improvise continuously, as if we were a jazz musician.

In our therapeutic as well as personal relationships, if we keep the awareness that we are always improvising, it infuses our interactions with much more liveliness and curiosity.

Throughout the session I want to be watching for working signs of the person's healthy response. Session design is as much about observation as plan, as much about listening with our whole self as communicating through touch. Much as in a jazz duet, one therapist/improviser will often attune half his focus to listening to the other!

In session design we are also practicing the scientific method. We make a hypothesis, experiment and measure our success, float a new hypothesis, test and re-measure, make new discoveries—on and on. In interviews before each session, I make "working assumptions" or "frames" based on what may be most relevant. I frame the session to match the most likely themes for our improvisation. However, the frame is no more the content of the session than the picture frame is the painting. If my working assumptions are fitting, it is more likely the client will show signs of positive response.

I am always trying to be conscious of and responsive to what I'm learning from that person. Indeed, while working I may find unexpectedly tense places; I may have new insights about how the person handles stress in their lives; I may see responses that cause me to question or refine my assumptions. That's fine—we are scientists and we are artists—we *want* to learn more! We *want* to sing the most beautiful song!

So much of this comes down to that beautiful phrase, "taking a history." Again may it be noted that while we may *give* a massage, we *take* or *receive* a history. Our gift to our client is to be truly interested in receiving the details needed to be of highest service to them! The gift for the therapist is to receive guidance from the client, who alone knows most deeply what s/he needs.

If I feel physically as if
the top of my head were taken off,
I know that is poetry.

— Emily Dickinson

Opening to inspiration

Even after thirty years of practice, often I am amazed that I still don't know what the outcome will be as I begin a session. I have high hopes, and some expectations, but I don't *know* what will happen. This is mostly good news. It creates within every session a unique context for wonder and surprise.

I may begin each session quietly with a fundamental prayer for guidance. I don't say it aloud, but I naturally think it. It centers me, and frames the session with the highest regard for the client, invoking the spiritual resources to work toward optimal therapeutic outcome. Like Emily Dickinson, you may feel the opening of your crown chakra as you invoke inspiration for your work together.

Looking

The second step of session design is to look with open eyes and really see the person. What is true for our client is true for all of us: we want to be seen and appreciated for who we most truly are. Let your mind, your associations, your whole self become receptive. Begin to develop a picture of this person in front of you and what their concerns may be.

Talking

I love the saying, "Don't talk unless you can improve on silence." Listen more than you speak. Listen with your whole self to what they say. Slight turns of phrase will reveal new facets of the gem that is your client.

Please respect and love the words you choose when conversing with your client. Well-chosen words on your part will facilitate the healing process for your client.

Listening

Taking a history is an invitation for the client to tell us their story. When you truly listen and hear their story, the clear, strong, and positive connection you receive is one of the great gifts of being a therapist.

Listen also to their tone of voice. Sometimes their words and tone are "syntonic," meaning they feel in harmony. Sometimes they're "dystonic," the tone and words apparently telling you two different things—when, for instance, someone might say he is happy, but his vocalization is infused with an opposing emotion that even his face may reveal.

Deeply Feeling

When a client opens up to you and you hear their story and its details—how they broke their arm; their rewarding study of martial arts; a childhood marked by moving every three years; the loss of a parent at an early age, the success in a career choice or the disappointment of a relationship gone awry—it is inevitable that your heart will open up. Truly hearing someone's story will awaken and evoke responsive feelings in you. These won't necessarily be feelings of empathy for their past injuries; they may equally be feelings of enthusiasm for the qualities and virtues this person displays.

In any case, please cultivate the ability to let your heart come to clarity about the themes most relevant for the person in this moment, and perhaps for the overall goals of therapy.

Emotional clarity will give rise to touch clarity. Remember, the most profound therapeutic changes are triggered by the client's neuroendocrine system. It in turn responds primarily to the feelings evoked by your touch. The clearer you are, the clearer they are. The more compassion you have for them, the more they will have for themselves.

Breathing

It's not enough merely to feel compassion. As a therapist it actually needs to flow into your hands. When you begin to have clarity about the feelings and themes relevant to your client, imagine breathing those messages through your whole body. Imagine that the frame, the themes for the session are expressed at the cellular level, through your entire body—not just your heart. This way every touch and every cell will convey relevant messages.

Sometimes, even with my best efforts, I may not come to any deep clarity about what is most relevant for a client on a given day. In that case, I just resolve to touch them at interface with highest personal regard, to manifest a high level of skill and care, and to leave space for the best outcome.

Get Excited

When I take a history, usually there is a point where the client and I are ready to stop talking and begin the session. It comes with excitement. Often it's the excitement of sensing what might be most helpful for the session about to begin. In any case, excitement arises because neither of us knows what will happen, although we both anticipate and hope for something helpful.

Stand Up!

As the session commences, I stand up and the client lies down. The act of standing is of course biomechanically necessary for Deep Massage. When we stand up, we stand beside this person. We stand for the triumph of their higher self, for their letting go of tension and pain, for them to have the energy and courage to fulfill their destiny.

Session Sequences

Over the course of a client's therapy, you will naturally vary each session to a greater or lesser degree. Here are some guidelines for putting together the work covered in the previous chapters.

1. Practice all the fulcrums in sequence so that you can do a full basic Deep Massage protocol in one hour.

2. For the first session, consider doing an entire Deep Massage protocol to get an overall feeling for the client and to give them an overall experience. In subsequent sessions, emphases will vary according to the client's individual nature, the presenting complaint(s) and the frame for the session.

3. In any case, in every session, do include the back and neck. Then, as called for,

emphasize other body areas: the legs, abdomen, shoulder girdle, pelvic girdle, etc. In advanced Deep Massage training, additional fulcrums are taught for the deeper muscles and for segments requiring more detailed hands-on instruction—for instance, iliopsoas, deeper neck muscles and ligaments, deeper rotators of the shoulder and hip, side-lying work, seated fulcrums, and the intrinsic muscles of the feet.

Ultimately, session design is a healing discussion carried on person-to-person, body-to-body. When we truly listen, our every action is informed by the truth of who the client is and who they may become. Trust that limitless benefits will flow from this.

BASIC DEEP MASSAGE PROTOCOL

Fists Down Erectors

Nine Points

Ironing Up Erectors

Levator Scapula

Posterior Neck – Trapezius, Semispinalis Capitis, Multifidus/Rotatores

Gluteus Maximus

Hamstrings

Gatrocnemius/Soleus

Tensor Fascia Lata, Gluteus Medius, and Gluteus Minimus

Iliotibial Band

Rectus Femoris

Peroneus Longus (aka "Fibularis")

Tibialis Anterior

Half Moon Vector through the Legs

Rectus Abdominis

Pectoralis Major

Biceps Brachii

Triceps Brachii

Trapezius (supine)

Scalenes

Facial Muscles

Epicranius

Half-Moon Vector through the Neck

Half-Moon Vector through the Legs

Everything Has an End

This might be the be-all and end-all — here…
Here, upon this bank and shoal of time, we'd jump the life to come.
— Shakespeare

Endings set the stage and create the room for new beginnings. The end for the seed is the new plant. From our hands at the ends of our arms, new creations continually spring forth.

This book is ending. I have loved every minute of writing it, even the struggles that accompany the process of all new things coming to life. It has been generating for over thirty years. What new beginnings will it provoke for you? My hope is that it facilitates your individual transformation, in turn helping the transformations of your clients, friends, family, and community. Everything you touch is affected by the deepest things you learn. Ultimately, everything we do issues into seeds of new worlds. From these spring forth growth in expected and unexpected ways.

When a session ends, we usually have no idea of how it will play out in a person's life. Months or even years later, a client or past student will often tell me a certain moment in a session or certain words spoken in a class changed their life. I had no idea! What tender and mysterious paths therapeutic actions and words take! I have the highest hopes for each person—for transformation or at least significant change—yet I don't know what the outcome will be.

When the session or class ends it is literally and figuratively out of our hands. I often feel a pang of loss—it is time to say goodbye. Equally I feel excitement and curiosity—what will the person make of it?

Goodbyes are less popular than hellos. They are often emotionally more complex.

Yet opportunity arises from the sacred art of ending. At the end of each session, each class, each book, new things come to life. We end with a sense of sacredness and mystery that naturally accompanies transition. Feelings of sadness, hope, exhaustion, awe, despair, curiosity, fear, elation, love, and serenity are natural. All these and more archetypically arise in the experience of ending. Let us choose that it end well and beautifully! As that movie, that symphony, that song, that class, that therapy session ends, may it leave a resonance reverberating positively in new ways for all our days.

Each Deep Massage can bring the person closer toward fulfilling their destiny. In each session, restraining forces introduced from previous experiences and locked into muscle, joint, bone, and nervous system are let go. We become freer; our natural inclination to grow, to enjoy, to live life to its fullest, is amplified. The present moment is now new, free, open to be lived as we please.

Each of us is a unique organism on the tree of life. We are influenced by our genes, the deep determining sap that shapes our body, mind, and spirit, going back ultimately to the very beginnings of life. We are influenced not only by our parents and their parents, but by our entire cultural and genetic heritage. We are the living repositories, for better and for worse, of ancestral qi. We are influenced by the events and decisions in our lives, consciously and unconsciously engendering our karma.

Every deep touch liberates the action potentials of our history. We are freer to be not only who we've been; we are freer to become who we are most truly. In this way, we are not mere objects or victims of our history. We have acquired a profound knowing: we are the subjects, the actors, and the creators of our unique history, of this world coming into each moment of being.

This tree of life, this giant wave of time and history, is vast and majestic for each individual and for all humankind, resplendent with every imaginable event and feeling. Our ancestors' dreams and lives do shape the world we inhabit. They have a claim; they have a stake in the realization of our common dreams. Through our lives and our living, they desire to see our deepest dreams realized—of peace, of freedom, of harmony. Many alive and many who have lived have suffered greatly; even now suffering around our globe calls out to us. People have triumphed and persevered through war and peace, love and hate, work and play. All the dreams of the past infuse our lives.

The history of humankind reveals restraining forces that need impede us no longer. War, selfish actions, environmental abuse, exploitation, and irrational hatreds, goaded by fear and ignorance, still play out among us. One philosopher said we will remain in the prehistory of humankind, the objects and victims of the past, until we become the subjects, the creators of our own present and future history.

Humans are unique in owning this capacity. No other animal can evolve in the span of a single lifetime; ordinarily it takes hundreds of generations. Humans have this incredibly precious capacity to learn and grow and change in fundamental ways so that one life, with all its changes, virtually becomes many lives.

What else is the point of life, but to optimize this opportunity? This uniquely human ability to evolve our being should be at the center of our education, our upbringing, even our politics.

The massage movement actually holds a key to accomplishing this transformation. Each part of our body has something vital to tell us about how we live. Since most parts of us don't speak in words, we need to listen to their deep language of pain, pleasure, intuition, feeling, and sensation. Therapists do this for a living, though we all can do it for a life!

History is not written in words but in actions. It is in the steps taken, the love felt, the decisions braved. It is in the breath that responds to each changing moment, the heart's promise, the opening to things and people, the exclamations of delight, the songs sung, the admiration of nature's myriad creations.

We live in the present moment, between the past with all its vast rivers of influence and the unknown future unfolding before us in all directions.

The interface of the present moment with what has passed and what is yet to come is where our work lies. The actions we take resonate back and forth through time, redeeming dreams of the past, transforming the present moment, and sowing the seeds of a healthier future.

Years ago, I did massage at a racquetball club in Chicago. I worked in a little basement room, next to the noisy weight room. One day, after a full schedule of therapy, I stepped into the glaring nightlights of northside Chicago and thought, *Oh, my God, am I going to be sixty years old and still doing this*? Then I saw that "The Karate Kid" was playing at a theater down the block. I went in. That film changed my life.

Particularly powerful for me was the moment when Mr. Miyagi, played beautifully by Pat Morita, is called upon to help the Karate Kid, who has badly sprained his ankle. Mr. Miyagi vigorously rubs his hands, claps forcefully, and places his hands on either side of the injured ankle. After this healing touch, Daniel-san, with a single lovely crane kick, overcomes his inner and outer opponent.

I emerged from the theater with the same thought in my head as when I entered, but with a completely new outlook.

The despair had been replaced by hope: *"Oh, my God, I'm still going to be doing this when I'm sixty. And by then, I'm going to be really good!"*

A study was done of the average time it takes for someone to achieve mastery in a complex psychomotor skill such as playing the piano. The average time is sixteen years! After more than thirty years in bodywork and fifty years in music, I am naturally humbled by how much I don't know. Remarkably, the path of mastery naturally includes recognizing just how much we have yet to master.

Whether you are a student, a massage therapist, other health practitioner, or general reader, may your dedication have the highest possible benefit for you and others. If you are not a health professional, I hope this book has enlightened you to the essential knowledge that is being brought forth through the expanding field of modern bodymind therapy.

What is it you will choose to do with your one wild and precious life?
— *Mary Oliver*

Have dedication and patience. Know that your work will result in transformations—sometimes when least expected, sometimes without us ever knowing they took place. This means every moment has transformative potential. This is what the great writer Walter Benjamin meant when he said, "Every second of time is the straight gate through which the Messiah might enter."

We cannot advance as a civilization if we do not recognize and harmonize with the highest contributions of our anatomy, physiology, and psychology. Progress based on technology and left brain logic alone is ultimately based on the loss of soul. Through the individual transformation of ourselves and others, I believe we can make as much progress spiritually and psychologically as we have technologically.

Given a mind that can envision infinite realities, an awareness of what we feel, and bodies of incredibly articulate action, let us choose and work hard to effect the highest possible positive impact.

Philosopher/writer Sam Keen once said, "Any question that you can answer in one lifetime is not a very good question." Similarly any end that we can accomplish in one lifetime is likely not a very lofty goal. The only exciting and fitting goal for the human experiment is to fulfill our potential, our ability to consciously create our reality, our best destiny—the conscious creation of peace on Earth.

The most important history is the one we make. Through our actions, with the work of our hands, we help create this new world. We facilitate the internal transformation of individuals. We help bring about world peace. It is the only way.

Although attempting to bring about
world peace through the internal
transformation of individuals is difficult,
it is the only way.

— H.H. Dalai Lama

Bibliography and Suggested Reading

ANATOMY AND PHYSIOLOGY

Biel, Andrew. *Trail Guide to the Body*. Boulder: Books of Discovery, 2010.

Clemente, Carmine. *Regional Atlas of Human Anatomy*. New York: Lippincott, Williams & Wilkins, 2006.

Dail, Nancy and Timothy Agnew. *Kinesiology for Manual Therapies*. New York: McGraw-Hill, 2011.

Strandring, Susan. *Gray's Anatomy*. (40th Edition) Philadelphia: Churchill Livingstone, 2009.

Kapandji, I.A, *Physiology of the Joints*. New York: Churchill Livingstone (3 vol.)1982.

Kapit, Wynn and Lawrence M. Elson. *Anatomy Coloring Book*. (3rd Edition) New Jersey: Benjamin Cummings, 2002.

Myers, Thomas. *Anatomy Trains*. New York: Churchill Livingstone, 2008.

Netter, Frank. *Atlas of Human Anatomy*. New York: Saunders/Elsevier 2006.

Platzer, Werner. *Color Atlas and Textbook of Human Anatomy: Locomotor System*. New York: Thieme Medical Publishers, 2004.

Rohen, Johannes W., Elke Lutjen-Drecoll, and Chichiro Yokochi. *Color Atlas of Anatomy*. New York: Lippincott Williams & Wilkins, 2010.

Tortora, Gerald J. and Nicholas P. Anagnostakos. *Principles of Anatomy and Physiology*. New York: Harper and Row, 1987.

PATHOLOGY

Salvo, Susan. *Mosby's Pathology for Massage Therapists*. New York: Mosby/Elsevier, 2008.

Werner, Ruth. *Massage Therapist's Guide to Pathology*. New York: Lippincott Williams & Wilkins, 2008.

NATURAL SCIENCE

Becker, Robert. *Body Electric*. New York: William Morrow and Company, 1985.

Bentov, Itzhak. *Stalking the Wild Pendulum*. New York: Bantam Books, 1977.

Capra, Fritjof. *Tao of Physics*. Boulder: Shambhala Publications, 1975.

Chopra, Deepak. *Quantum Healing*. New York: Bantam Books, 1990.

Field, Tiffany. *Touch*. Cambridge, MA: The MIT Press, 2003.

Juhan, Dean. *Job's Body*. Barrytown, NY: Station Hill Press, 2003.

Montagu, Ashley. *Touching: The Human Significance of the Skin*. New York: Harper and Row, 1971.

Murphy, Michael. *The Future of the Body*. New York: J.P.Tarcher, 1992.

_____. *Jacob Atabet*. New York: J.P.Tarcher, 1988.

Oschman, James. *Energy Medicine*. New York: Churchill Livingstone, 2000.

Rossi, Ernest. *Psychobiology of Mind-Body Healing*. New York: W.W. Norton and Company, 1993.

Schwenk, Theodor. *Sensitive Chaos*. London: Rudolf Steiner Press, 1996.

Simeons, A. T. W. *Man's Presumptuous Brain*. New York: E.P. Dutton, 1960.

MASSAGE AND BODYWORK

Benjamin, Ben. *Listen to Your Pain*. New York: Penguin Group, 2007.

Benjamin, P. and S. Lamp. *Understanding Sports Massage*. Champagne, IL: Human Kinetics, 2004.

Chaitow, Leon. *Soft Tissue Manipulation*. Rochester, VT: Healing Arts Press, 1988.

Cottingham, John. *Healing Through Touch*. Boulder, CO.: Rolf Inst., 1985.

Downing, George. *The Massage Book*. New York: Random House, 1998.

_____. *Massage and Meditation*. New York: Random House, 1974.

Earls, James and Thomas Myers. *Fascial Release for Structural Balance*, Berkeley, CA.: North Atlantic Books, 2011.

Johnson, Don. *The Protean Body*. New York: Harper and Row, 1977.

Kunz, Kevin and Barbara. *Complete Guide to Foot Reflexology*. New York, 1980.

Lauterstein, David. *Putting the Soul Back in the Body*. Chicago: 1984.

_____. "What is Zero Balancing?" Massage Therapy Journal, Winter 1994: pp. 28-35.

Lundberg, Paul. *Book of Shiatsu*. New York: Simon and Schuster, 1992, 2014.

McClure, Vimala. *Infant Massage: A Handbook for Loving Parents*. New York: Bantam Books, 2000.

Milne, Hugh. *Heart of Listening*. Berkeley, CA: North Atlantic Books, 1995.

Ohashi, W. *Do-It-Yourself Shiatsu*. New York: Penguin Books, 2001.

Osborne-Sheets, Carole. *Deep Tissue Sculpting*. San Diego: Body Therapy Associates, 1990.

Rattray, F. and L. Ludwig. *Clinical Massage Therapy: Understanding, Assessing and Treating Over 70 Conditions*. West Vancouver, Canada: Talus, 2005.

Rolf, Ida. *Rolfing and Physical Reality*. Rochester, VT: Healing Arts Press, 1990.

_____. *Rolfing*. Rochester, VT: Healing Arts Press, 1989.

Salvo, Susan. *Massage Therapy: Principles and Practice*. New York: Elsevier, 2011.

Sinclair, Marybetts. *Pediatric Massage Therapy*. Philadelphia: Lippincott Williams & Wilkins, 2005.

Smith, Fritz Frederick. *Inner Bridges*. Lake Worth, FL: Humanics, 1986.

_____. *Alchemy of Touch*. Taos, NM: Complementary Medicine Press, 2005.

Smith, John. *Structural Bodywork*. New York: Elsevier, 2005.

Stone, Randolph. *Polarity Therapy*. (two volumes) Summertown, TN: Book Pub Co., 1999.

Tappan, Frances. *Tappan's Handbook of Healing Massage Techniques*. New York: Pearson, 2009.

Travell, Janet. *Myofascial Pain and Dysfunction*. (2 vols.) Philadelphia: Lippincott Williams and Wilkins, 1993.

Teeguarden, Iona. *Joy of Feeling: Bodymind Accupressure*. Idyllwild, CA: Jin Shin Do Foundation, 2006.

Upledger, John. *Craniosacral Therapy*. Berkeley: North Atlantic Books, 2001.

MOVEMENT SKILLS AND SELF-CARE

Anderson, Bob. *Stretching*. Bolinas, CA: Shelter Publications, 1980.

Feldenkrais, Moshe. *Awareness Through Movement*. New York: Harper and Row, 1972.

_____. *Body and Mature Behavior*. Berkeley: Frog Books, 2005.

Greene, Lauriann and Richard Goggins. *Save Your Hands: The Complete Guide to Injury Prevention and Ergonomics for Manual Therapists*. Coconut Creek, FL: Body of Work Books, 2008.

Ichazo, Oscar. *Arica Psychocalisthenics*. New York: Simon and Schuster, 1976.

Lowen, Alexander. *Way to Vibrant Health*. Alachua, FL: Bioenergetics Press, 2003.

Mattes, Aaron. *Flexibility for Conditioning and Rehabilitation*. Mattes, 1980.

Olson, Andrea. *Bodystories*. Barrytown, NY: Station Hill, 1998.

Todd, Mabel Elsworth. *The Thinking Body*. New York: Paul Hoeber, Inc. 1937.

NUTRITION, HERBS AND NATURAL LIVING

Ballentine, Rudolph. *Diet and Nutrition*. Honesdale, PA: Himalayan Institute Press, 1978.

Haas, Elson. *Staying Healthy with the Seasons*. Berkeley, CA: Ten Speed Press, 2004.

Ladd, Vasant. *Ayurveda: The Science of Self-Healing*. Twin Lakes, WI: Lotus Press, 2004.

_____. *Yoga of Herbs*. Twin Lakes, WI: Lotus Press, 1992.

Lipski, Elizabeth. *Digestive Wellness*. New York: McGraw-Hill, 2005.

McCamy, John and James Presley. *Human Life-Styling*. New York: HarperCollins Publishers, 1978.

Kirschman, John. *Nutrition Almanac*. New York: McGraw-Hill, 2007.

Thrash, Agatha. *Home Remedies : Hydrotherapy, Massage Charcoal, and Other Simple Treatments*. Seale, AL: New Lifestyle Books, 1981.

Tierra, Michael. *The Way of Herbs*. New York: Simon and Schuster, 1998.

Tisserand, Robert. *Aromatherapy to Heal and Tend the Body*. Twin Lakes, WI: Lotus Press, 1988.

ENERGETIC HEALING

Brennan, Barbara. *Hands of Light*. New York: Bantam Books, 1988.

Castenada, Carlos. *Journey to Ixtlan*. New York: Simon and Schuster, 1972.

Gerber, Richard. *Vibrational Medicine*. Rochester, VT: Bear and Co., 1996.

Harner, Michael. *Way of the Shaman*. New York: HarperCollins Publishers, 1990.

Lamb, Bruce. *Wizard of the Upper Amazon*. Berkeley, CA: North Atlantic Books, 1986.

ASIAN MEDICINE

Chia, Mantak. *Awaken Healing Energy through the Tao*. Santa Fe, NM: Aurora Press, 1983.

Connelly, Diane. *Traditional Acupuncture: The Law of the Five Elements*. Columbia, MD: Traditional Acupuncture Institute, 1994.

Kaptchuk, Ted. *Web That Has No Weaver*. New York: McGraw-Hill, 2000.

Larre, Claude and Elisabeth Rochat de la Vallee. *Rooted in the Spirit*. Barrytown, NY: Station Hill Press, 1995.

Legge, David. *Close To The Bone*. Woy Woy, Australia: Sydney College Press, 2000.

Masunaga, Shizuto. *Zen Imagery Exercises*. Tokyo: Japan Publications, 1987.

Veith, Ilza. *Yellow Emperor's Classic of Internal Medicine*. Berkeley, CA: University of California Press, 1972.

MEDITATION/ SPIRITUALITY

Anon. *New American Standard Bible*. La Habra, CA: Foundation Publications, 1997.

Dass, Ram. *Be Here Now*. New York: HarperCollins Publishers, 1971.

Hanh, Thich Nat. *Peace is Every Step*. New York: Bantam Books, 1991.

Lao Tsu. *Tao Te Ching*. New York: Vintage Books, 1997.

Merton, Thomas. *New Seeds of Contemplation*. New York: New Directions Publishing, 2007.

Suzuki, Shunryu. *Zen Mind, Beginner's Mind*. Boston: Weatherhill, 1973.

Trungpa, Chogyam. *Cutting Through Spiritual Materialism*. Boston: Shambhala Publications, 1973.

Weil, Simone. *Gravity and Grace*. New York: Routledge, 1987.

Wilhelm, Hellmut. *I Ching*. Princeton, NJ: Princeton University Press, 1973.

PHILOSOPHY, POETRY, AND LITERATURE OF HEALING

Benjamin, Walter. *Illuminations*. New York: Schocken Books, 1969.

Berger, John. *Selected Writings*. New York: Pantheon, 2001.

Bernanos, George. *Diary of a Country Priest*. New York: Carroll and Graf Publishers (Avalon Publishing Group), 2002.

Blake, Willliam. *The Marriage of Heaven and Hell*. New York: Oxford University Press, 1975.

Buber, Martin. *Between Man and Man*. New York: Macmillan Publishing Co., 1965.

Bloomer, Kent and Charles Moore. *Body, Memory and Architecture*. New Haven, CT: Yale University Press, 1977.

Bly, Robert. *News of the Universe*. San Francisco: Sierra Club Books, 1995.

Campbell, Joseph. *The Mythic Image*. Princeton, NJ: Princeton University Press, 1974.

Dickinson, Emily. *Complete Poems of Emily Dickinson.* Boston: Back Bay Books, 1976.

Hesse, Herman. *Siddhartha.* New York: Bantam Classics, 1981.

Hyde, Lewis. *The Gift.* New York: Vintage, 1979.

Lusseyran, Jacques. *And There Was Light.* Sandpoint, ID: Morning Light Press, 1998.

Mitchell, Stephen. *The Enlightened Heart.* New York: HarperCollins Publishers, 1989.

Neruda, Pablo. *Residence on Earth.* New York: New Directions, 1973.

Nye, Naomi. *Words under the Words.* Portland, OR: Far Corner Books, 1995.

Rilke, Rainer Maria. *Letters to a Young Poet.* New York: W. W. Norton, 1993.

Rumi Jelaluddin and Coleman Barks. *Delicious Laughter.* Athens, GA: Maypop, 1990.

Tsunetomo, Yamamoto. *Hagakure: Book of the Samurai.* New York: Kodansha International, 1983.

Vallejo, Cesar. *Poemas Humanos.* New York: Grove Press, 1968.

Whitman, Walt. *Leaves of Grass.* New York: Eakins Press, 1966.

POLITICS AND HISTORY

Calvert, Robert. *History of Massage.* Rochester, VT: Healing Arts Press, 2002.

Ehrenreich, B. and D. English. *Witches, Midwives and Nurses.* New York: Feminist Press, 2010.

Gevitz, Norman. *Other Healers: Unorthodox Medicine in America.* Baltimore, MD: Johns Hopkins University Press, 1988.

Illich, Ivan. *Medical Nemesis.* New York: Random House, 1976.

Zweig, Stefan. *Mental Healers.* New York: Frederick Ungar Publishing Co., 1962

PSYCHOLOGY

Erickson, Milton. *My Voice Will Go with You.* New York: W. W. Norton, 1991.

Gendlin, Eugene. *Focusing.* New York: Bantam Books, 1982.

Green, E. and B. Goodrich-Dunn. *Psychology of the Body.* New York: Lippincott, Williams & Wilkins, 2004.

Haldane, S. *Emotional First Aid.* Barrytown, NY: Station Hill Press, 1998.

Johnson, Robert. *Ecstasy.* New York: HarperCollins Publishers, 1987.

Keleman, Stanley. *Emotional Anatomy.* Thousand Oaks, CA: Center Press, 1985.

Kopp, Sheldon. *If You Meet the Buddha on the Road, Kill Him*. New York: Bantam Books, 1982.

Kubler-Ross, Elizabeth. *On Death and Dying*. New York: Simon and Schuster, 1997.

Kurtz, Ron. *Body-Centered Psychotherapy*. Mendocino, CA: LifeRhythm, 2007.

Laing, R.D. *The Divided Self*. New York: Routledge, 2001.

———. *The Politics of Experience*. New York: Penguin Books, 1990.

Lowen, Alexander. *Language of the Body*. Alachua, FL: Bioenergetics Press, 2006.

Moore, Thomas. *Care of the Soul*. New York: HarperCollins Publishers, 1994.

Perls, F. Ego, *Hunger and Aggression*. New York: Vintage, 1969.

Perls, F., R. Hefferline, and P. Goodman. *Gestalt Therapy*. Gouldsboro, ME: Gestalt Journal Press, 2005.

Reich, Wilhelm. *Character Analysis*. New York: Farrar, Straus and Giroux, 1972.

———. *Function of the Orgasm*. New York: Noonday Press, 1961.

Welwood, John. *Challenge of the Heart*. Boston: Shambhala Publications, 1985.

BUSINESS AND ETHICS

Abraham, Jay. *Getting Everything You Can out of All You've Got*. New York: St. Martin's Griffin, 2000.

Bolles, Richard. *What Color is Your Parachute?* Berkeley, CA: Ten Speed Press, 2011.

Covey, Stephen. *The Seven Habits of Highly Effective People*. New York: Free Press, 2004.

Hawken, Paul. *Growing a Business*. New York: Simon and Schuster, 1987.

Palmer, David. *The Bodywork Entrepreneur*. New York: Thumb Press, 1990.

Phillips, Michael and Salli Rasberry. *Marketing without Advertising*. Berkeley, CA: Nolo Press, 2003.

Sohnen-Moe, Cherie. *Business Mastery*. Tucson, AZ: Sohnen-Moe Associates, 2007.

———, and Ben E. Benjamin. *Ethics of Touch*. Tucson, AZ: Sohnen-Moe Associates, 2003.

Index

rotatores, 50, 158, 166, *170-171*
Rumi, 133, 155

S

sacrum, 52-53, 127
sadness, 165
satyagraha, 84
Save Your Hands, 39
scalene muscles, 36, 158, 163, 165-166
scalenes, 164
scapula, 50, 60
self-esteem issues, 165
self-imaging of body structure, 82
self-realization, 182
semimembranosus, 74-76
semispinalis, 158, 166, 168, 169, *170*
sensori-motor amnesia, 58, 88
Sessions, Roger, 63
seven dimensions of touch, 44, 177-178
Shakespeare, William 193
shoulder girdle, 50, 93, 114, 124, 127, 132-133, 145, 190
sitz bones, 74, 76
Smith, Fritz, vi, 67
somatic transformation, 178
spinal compression, 50
spinal cord, 114
spinalis, 50, 166
spinous process, 50
spirit, 6, 9-12, 14-15, 17, 26, 28, 35, 47-48, 62, 80-82, 85, 87, 102, 111, 127-130, 148-154, 156, 174, 177
sports massage, 64, 79
staying at interface, 47
sternocleidomastoid, 158, 165
Still, Andrew Taylor, 4, 43, 48, 110, 180
strengthening exercises for massage therapists, 39
stress, 4, 30, 50, 140, 142, 144-146, 180
stretch reflex, 67
suboccipital muscles, 158

substance addictions, 180
supination of the ankle, 88
supraspinatus, 60
supraspinous fossa, 60
sustaining the gesture, 16, *21*
Suzuki, Shunryu, 21
swallowing as parasympathetic response, 30
Swedish massage, 3, 37, 40, 42, 62
sympathetomimetic hormones, 179

T

T1, 60, 170
T11, 58
T12, 166
T7, 60
T8, 60
tai chi, 39, 107
take out the looseness, 16, *18-19*
Taking up the slack, 16, 19
T-cells, 125
temporal energy flow, 150
temporal integration, 150
temporalis, 158
temporoparietalis, 158
tendons, 5
tensegrity, 4
tension, 14, 18-19, 27, 29, 40, 47, 51, 54, 58, 60, 66, 82, 88-89, 102, 104, 110-111, 115-116, 129, 132, 145-146, 155, 157, 166, 190
tensor fascia lata, 36, 92-93, *94*, 95
therapeutic hypocracy, 47
therapist's emotions during a session, 47
thixotrophic, 6, 66, 110
thoracic health and fullness of breath, 51
Thoreau, Henry David, 126
throat chakra, 128
thymus gland, 125
tibialis anterior, 36, 100, *101*
Tillinghast, Richard, 157

touch, evolutionary role of, 12
touch, energetic and structural quality, 13
touch, seven dimensions of, 35
Trager, Milton, 151
transformations, 196
trapezius, 36, 50-52, 60, 124, 142, *143*, 144-146, 158, 166, *167*, 168
trauma from childhood, 124
triceps brachii, 36, 138-*139*

U

understanding, 178
universal life flow, 172

V

vastus intermedius, 89
verbal feedback during massage session, 29
voice vitality, 28

W

weight training, 39
whiplash, 165
Whitman, Walt, 67
Wittgenstein, Ludwig, 178
working at interface, 13-14, 46
working breath cycle, 28
working sign, 22, 25-30, 91
working state, 25-26

Y

yoga, 39, 107

Z

Zen meditation, 39
Zen tradition, 149
Zero Balancing, iii-iv, vi, 3, 28, 42, 107, 166, 182, 185, 201